# About the Author

Catherine Baker was born in the East End of postwar London. Her mother called her the "elderly baby", and her father once told her, "I don't know where *you* came from".

Driven by the feeling that she didn't belong, Catherine moved through several continents and personas before "coming home" to the fertile beauty of eastern Australia. She now lives close to the land in northern NSW, working as a teacher and writer, and forever intrigued by the horrors, the joys and the mysteries of life.

# RINGING
# THE
# CHANGE

To the Venerable Sangharakshita, who has said:

*Between male and female there will always be war, or at least tension. The only solution is for both men and women to try to develop both "masculine" and "feminine" qualities within themselves and relate to one another as individuals.*

# RINGING
# THE
# CHANGE

## CATHERINE
## BAKER

**DOUBLEDAY**

SYDNEY • AUCKLAND • TORONTO • NEW YORK • LONDON

RINGING THE CHANGE
A DOUBLEDAY BOOK

First published in Australia and New Zealand
in 1996 by Doubleday

National Library of Australia
Cataloguing-in-Publication Entry

Baker, Catherine, 1944– .
    Ringing the change : a journey of self-discovery.

    ISBN 0 86824 646 8.

    1. Baker, Catherine, 1944–  . –Diaries. 2. Divorced women–
    Biography. 3. Menopause–Psychological aspects. I. Title.

306.89

Doubleday books are published by

Transworld Publishers (Aust) Pty Limited
15–25 Helles Ave, Moorebank, NSW 2170

Transworld Publishers (NZ) Limited
3 William Pickering Drive, Albany, Auckland

Transworld Publishers (UK) Limited
61–63 Uxbridge Road, Ealing, London W5 5SA

Bantam Doubleday Dell Publishing Group Inc
1540 Broadway, New York, New York 10036

Cover design by Reno Design Group (15019)
Cover painting *Nerissa* by John William Godward
Text design by Anaconda Graphic Design
Production by Vantage Graphics
Typeset in Cochin Regular by Midland Typesetters, Victoria
Printed by Australian Print Group, Victoria

10 9 8 7 6 5 4 3 2 1

# Contents

# Acknowledgements

The author and publisher would like to acknowledge the following sources:

Charlotte Joko Beck, *Everyday Zen*, Harper and Row, Publishers Inc., 1989. (Copyright Charlotte Joko Beck and Steve Smith.) Extract reproduced with the permission of HarperCollins USA.

Annie Dillard, *The Writing Life*, Harper Perennial, 1989.

Germaine Greer, *The Change*, Hamish Hamilton/Penguin Group, 1991.

Robert Hand, *Planets in Transit*, Schiffer Publishing Ltd, 1976.

Janet Hawley, "An Imaginary Life" (interview with David Malouf), *Good Weekend* magazine, 27 March 1993. Extract reproduced with the permission of the *Good Weekend*.

Marc Robertson, *Transit of Saturn: Critical Ages in Adult Life*, American Federation of Astrologers, 1976. Extracts reproduced with the permission of the publishers.

# An Introduction

*Do I contradict myself?*
*Very well then, I contradict myself.*
*I am large, I contain multitudes.*

Walt Whitman
*Song of Myself*

I was born of that generation of women that cried at *Gone With the Wind*. That found the marital rape scene romantic. My three paper-nylon petticoats stiff beneath my Bo-Peep skirt shifted secretly among themselves as my thighs tightened in response to the incorrigible Rhett Butler bounding up that staircase two steps at a time with the struggling Scarlett in his manly arms.

I swooned in anticipation of something similar happening to me. I was about twelve, or perhaps thirteen. It was about 1956, or 1957. *Gone With the Wind* had never stopped playing somewhere in the world and adults had never stopped imposing their romantic aspirations upon children.

Romantic means remote from experience. So the adult ruling that "between our legs" was a place to be ignored except for hygiene was also rather romantic, being an idea remote from the experience of most children. For us, "between our legs" was a source of endless conjecture. When would *we* be allowed to taste those Hollywood games?

There is no blame here. Some forms of meaning eluded our parents and teachers just as certain other forms elude we parents and teachers. Like most children, I felt love for my parents without needing to understand them. But that kind of wisdom was lost in the seas of my first adulthood. It is re-surfacing now, now that I am fifty. And now that I am fifty, I see my parents' reluctance to draw my attention

to the functions of the female parts as testimony to their
human-ness. They were not . . . what we become conditioned
to expect from our loved ones . . . they were not . . . perfect.

Looking through the windows of my past from a
perspective over half-way through my life, I see more
clearly the Anglo-Saxon silence about female mysteries. I
see the shame, the ignorance that littered our puberty and
still clutters our path into "the youth of our second
adulthood", as a friend has described her menopause.

The first hint that there were mysteries connected with
bits of my body came to me when I was about seven years
old. It was when my father stopped helping me dry myself
after bathtime. "You're old enough to do it by yourself
now", he said darkly. Then he added, in even shadier
terms, "And don't forget to dry between your legs".

I took "between my legs" with all the *esprit de corps* of
the child, towelling extra hard from the inside of my thigh
to the inside of my knee and down, down, down to the
mysterious inside of my ankle. Puzzled though I was that
my inside-leg should suddenly take on such significance,
the once-a-week cleansing ritual in our old tin bath out
back in the scullery was religiously rounded off in this way
for the next few years. Both legs.

I didn't go near my vagina. Nobody had mentioned *that*.
Nobody ever did mention *that*. And being a cerebral child
(and still, alas, to some extent a cerebral adult), needing
words in order to respond to reality, my fingers never did
hasten with libidinous frivolity towards my clitoris. Nobody
had ever told me it was *there*. Or perhaps they had, earlier
than memory can take me. And perhaps they had told me
that fingers down there got dirty, nasty, bad, and slapped
them away, as I later saw happening to my friends' younger
sisters.

It wasn't until I was about eleven, in fact, that my bold
girlfriend Yvonne leapt the barricades of decorum and
dragged my mind below the level of my eyebrows. "It's

called yer virginia", she told me, "an' if somefink gets put innit, it can split yer right up the middle!"

In the East End of post-war London I held tight my childhood wisdom, that child's sense which accepts things as they are, amid the hopelessness bred by our poverty. My parents' dreams of wealth and staircases like Rhett Butler's made their lives hard, harder than if poverty dwells only with itself, where there are no aspirations. They saved up their shillings for the gas meter, made sacrifices for their children, hurt with love for their children, and refused to budge on the inconceivable, the miraculous, the prodigious and absurd fundamentals of existence. I looked up at our meagre share of the stars and felt an anguish of separation, of utter puzzlement. When I asked my mother if babies came "just from the forsation of love" (another of Yvonne's linguistic errors), she averted her eyes and said, embarrassed, "You'll find out".

I had known long before then that I had been born in the wrong place. Its heavy-water skies bent me double, wrapped stifling layers of clothing around my heart-stories of sun-warmed horizons moving against crimson skies. In the huge Australian glasshouse at Kew Gardens, my dreams expanded in the heat; I smiled at the leaf-shapes; I smelled a memory much older than myself.

The land ran through that memory. The land, the sky, the trees, the animals. Not just people, and buses, and streets. I told the flame-haired Margaret O'Toole, whose arithmetic work I used to copy, "I'm gonna live in Australia when I grow up. I'm gonna live on a farm". Australia not being part of the Known World in 1956, or 1957, Margaret replied, "Wot yer wanna go there for? That's where Adolf 'itler wos bawn!"

At my all-girls "technical" high school, we cooked and sewed and learned more about adult embarrassment during the lessons called "hygiene", a word that in my unharnessed mind ran alongside wire-brushes and carbolic soap. An appropriate image indeed for the naughty daughters of Eve.

The heaving booming hygiene teacher, Miss Bell, had one truth. It was the male truth of science. It was the biology of the thing. Limited, very limited, biology. I have since known biologists who give themselves pilots' licences to take their students on poetic word-flights of epic proportions around the peaks and into the valleys of sperm meeting egg. But Miss Bell had us all keep company with her thunderous and virginal self in the hangar of ignorance. And as one fine writer has put it, what can a virgin possibly know of the travails of humanity?

Sperm got a hurried acknowledgement. It was all alone. Testicles, penises and penetration went unremarked. Uterus, eggs and fallopian tubes merited a diagram in our books. Blood was touched upon. And the Devil take those girls who didn't keep themselves clean.

There was no mention of what puberty might mean to us spiritually, psychologically, sexually. There was no mention of the responsibilities, the joys and the trials of forty years of fertility. And there was no mention of the Change—the fragile threshold on which I currently stand.

There was nothing for us from the heart, nothing from life. There was only the shame of it. And still no-one had verified for me whether penetration of the vagina (I had the right word now) really did split you up the middle.

Understanding that this ghastly image was a scare tactic designed to protect young girls of the Empire from sin finally dawned with rabbits. There were diagrams of their disembodied sex organs "doing it" in our biology books. Rumour ran rife. It was hinted that that was how *we* do it too. I finally confirmed the truth of this horror in the public library, guardedly, slinking between the shelves of the adult science section. I was with my friend Claudette. We were thunderstruck. "D'you mean ..." I remember shrilling to her, not expecting any kind of answer, "D'you mean the

Queen and the Jook of Edinburgh do *that*?"

Now I was ready with a further question for my mother. "Wossit like, Mum, makin' luv wiv a man?"

She looked aside at the wallpaper, defied me to trouble her further by saying in unequivocal tones, "It's 'orrible!"

To such an extent we had learned to revile our bodies. And it wasn't just in the East End. It was Empire-wide. We wartime girls found our curiosity and imaginations blocked on all sides by paranoia about the sinfulness of sex and essential corruptness of the body.

So by the time menstruation came our minds had been made sordid by behind-the-hand references to "sanitary towels", "sanitary belts", and "sanitary pins" big enough for a baby's nappy. We did not welcome the flux, the menses, did not see it as the beginning or ending of anything significant. Saw it only as dirty, painful, shameful.

When my sister, three years older than me, first "came on", I had covered my eyes with my hands as she and my mother flurried about with unmentionable paraphernalia. "I won't look! I won't look!" I promised, having come upon them by surprise, to save my sister's tears. And I kept my promise. However, I considered myself trained in the matter, and when my turn came, I did not seek my mother's help. Weakly and with distaste, I went about the necessary "business".

It came again. And again. And again. With no apparent connection to anything else. The moon? I could not see it for the rooftops. My mother could not see it for the rooftops. Miss Bell could not see it for the rooftops.

Boys? Men? What were they? Certainly not my father. He was my father. I had no brothers. Cousins, yes. But they were not boys or men either. They were my cousins.

Boys and men could—possibly—be Rhett Butler, or Clark Gable if you were more pragmatic. Which meant they had to look good. In accordance with Hollywood Principles. That was all that mattered.

Furnished with this paltry guideline we grew breasts and launched ourselves like lemmings into the big seas of our sexuality. "Saw yer wiv yer boyfriend last night", said a cheeky child in a younger class, when I was seventeen and stepping out with a twenty-year-old "artist" who gave me my first kiss-on-the-mouth. "I reckon 'e's smashin'", she concluded. Well, you should have seen me puff up. Having a boyfriend was a symbol of being just a regular girl, one who shared the dreams and fancies of her schoolmates.

The wintry kisses against the frost-laden walls of West Ham Football Ground aroused nothing in me but words, ideas, associations. I wanted to talk, to lift us out of the bombed sites and concerns for our "love" to a place my heart had refused to let go; a "child's" place if you like, a bizarre playground unconcerned with the adult way of thinking-in-a-straight-line-from-past-to-present-to-golden-future.

"We could get married", the twenty-year-old looker suggested once or twice.

Get married? Why would I want to do that cosy-for-life thing? Its legalities left no room for contradiction, for change. Marriage had no appeal. The closeness of couples with their children in the little terraced houses of West Ham brought forth no longing, nothing to change what I instinctively knew: that the very process of life was the enemy of such plans, made when one was so young. He was offended. "I've already had a trial marriage", he protested, "I'm not young."

Contrary to working-class expectation, I was accepted for university. I was one of the first two hopefuls from my once technical, but recently turned grammar, school. Hesitant, I now found myself sitting in lectures on equal terms with boys, rather big boys. My eyes bored into the backs of the handsome ones' heads, only to be quickly averted should they turn around and catch me. Oh brave new world that had such creatures in it! I drafted fantasies of lying with them in wheatfields wearing only a bra and knickers and a full-length petticoat and a thin summer frock that showed my long creamy neck to perfection . . . and oh, how we would talk!

In my dreams they never groped me. Nor in reality either. These were English dreams, this was English reality, these were English boys, and it was 1963. I eventually lay with Bob (third-year student, Beatle Jacket, winkle-picker boots), not in any sort of wheatfield, but in my chill back-room of the house I rented with three other girls in Loughborough Road, Leicester. They, too, had boyfriends that they lay with. But none of us, yet, was actually "doing it". Possible pregnancy loomed large in our asexual legend. That much we agreed.

What we never discussed — and this is testimony to the times — was whether we really *wanted* to "do it". There was an unspoken general agreement that sure, yeah, sure, we're sexy aren't we? We'd love to do it, but . . .

God entered neither my bedroom nor that still point in my heart where all other points came together. That point where, on those rare occasions when it revealed itself to me, I could sit and see and listen to . . . not the ethics of hypocritical sanctions, but the ethics of inner reference. This ethic arose from a sense of personal strength, a sense of "alrightness" within; an admittedly dim light which had to do with the Buddhist symbol of the lotus flower . . . of fragrant beauty blossoming from mud. A symbol that lay quietly for many years before stirring in my story.

It was nice and harmless lying with Bob; homely on cold nights, separated by flannel nightie and pyjamas. He'd had one previous encounter, had "gone all the way" with a girl known around town as Horizontal, told me it was "a bit of a shock really". He had an idea about marrying me and was prepared to wait.

We kissed and cuddled. I seem to remember him fondling

my breasts. But below the belt was out-of-bounds. I'd still had no contact with my own vagina, had no real idea how it might be angled in those forbidden folds, so I was damned if I was going to let any outsider touch it. As for the male organ—completely uncharted. My incurious fingers neither touched nor cared to touch. If Bob ever had an erection while lying beside me and kissing, it failed to get my attention. Perhaps because "erection", like "clitoris", was not a word I knew. They were not yet part of common parlance.

So it went for a year or so. During which time one of my flatmates admitted to blazing the forbidden trail with her almost-fiancé. "What's it like?" I asked her. (University education had helped me revise my Cockney accent.) "It's alright", she said, clearly wishing to add nothing more. I could tell it was not "alright". But the matter was closed due to embarrassment. This was my closest friend.

And then ... And then ...

Ah! On the ship to Africa, rolling in the Bay of Biscay, I tensed myself against the toilet wall, took an unfamiliar Tampax from its unfamiliar packet, fumbled the applicator into some sort of position, and discovered my vagina.

My amazement at how easy, how smooth, how slippery-eel it was, once you knew where. I almost leapt in the air for the absolute ease and comfort of it. So that was where penises got put! It did not hurt at all! Holy Mary Mother of God, this is half-way revolutionary!

And so it was, for me. The packet of Tampax I had purchased just before leaving England was in my mind a passport to sunbathing all-month-round. I had not imagined that the no-more bulky-sanitary-towels decision would lead me to a series of men that did more than fondle and wait for me to marry them. But this hygienic and practical determination was in fact a big part of the picture.

Another was the Pill. Now that I knew where my vagina was, I wanted to experiment. The Indian doctor that made the Pill available to me admonished me about getting married eventually, and I said yes, yes, yes, of course. And away I went.

I would not say that it did not matter which man it was, but it could have been any one of, say, half a dozen, in our elite group of sixty newly-graduated Englishpersons shipped out to East Africa by the then Ministry of Overseas Development to bring academic enlightenment to African high school students. It was 1965. I was twenty-one years old. And I had a suntan.

I chose the one that made me laugh the most. Fortunately he'd had some previous experience. I pretended that I had too, and I groaned a little, dug my nails in his back because I had read that was what passionate women did. I think I faked well because he never said anything that suggested he thought me a phoney. Though I was unimpressed by the experience, I do recall a brief moment of engagement, when I thought, "Oh, this is quite nice", but then suddenly it was over. Anti-climax would be an appropriate description. The act remained a curiosity. My strictly-missionary-position lover's indulgences remained just something that men did.

What mattered was that now I was no longer a virgin. A sense of pride in this accompanied my post-sex bath in the prosaic grey washblock of our trainee teachers' residence. We did it again a few days later; this time it was I who climbed in through *his* window and he made me giggle by telling jokes in Latin. By my choice, we left our carnal knowledge of one another at that. Each found other lovers. We remained great friends, and it was not until many years later that he told me he had never understood how — or why — the passion came and went so quickly. Even then, when I was — what, twenty-eight? — and it was 1972, I was still too abashed by the whole sorry topic to admit to him that at the time I just needed his dear self with his gentle ways and sense of the absurd to breach my virginal walls.

But I had learned enough about myself in those first few years out of England to realise that I liked the men I knew, relished their company, relished the exchange of ideas. That they were so interested in establishing possible rules by which things functioned was in no way a threat to my female intuitiveness on similar matters. My child's heart still held that "the universe shakes and trembles and sits different ways", as I read years later in the Buddhist *White Lotus Sutra*. And my men friends' laboratory-tested thinking was just one of those ways of sitting, affording me endless mind-games.

Listen: If at the sub-atomic level all events are governed only by probabilities rather than hard-and-fast physical laws, as shown again and again in the laboratories of quantum physicists, *events at all levels must be governed only by probabilities*. Even though at our everyday level of buses and bread and boys, the sum total of those sub-atomic probabilities looks no different from what we understand to be hard-and-fast physical laws.

So, if basic phenomena are governed only by probabilities—which I had suspected all along anyway, but now they were telling me it was *proven*—how could anybody possibly be dogmatic? Yet people *were*! People *are*! Dogmatic about almost everything! About who should love who, about who should marry who, about what makes a marriage, about what makes a family, about what to expect from one another, about what we deserve from life, about what makes us happy and how to hold onto it, about what makes us sad and how to avoid it, about what opinions we should stick to in order to get certain results, and so on and so on.

When I was growing up, while others were telling me to hold on to my slippery opinions, to try to keep hold of a happiness that came and went and came and went, to steer clear of pain (that would of course eventually have to be faced), the probable-ness in my heart crouched and diminished for lack of shelter. Now though, this male science, born of equations pencilled on table-tops in cafes in Austria and Germany, gave my probable-ness a roof over its head. Gave a respectable home to my still point, where for years I had sat and breathed in paradox. The scientifically-proven probable-ness of the universe confirmed my sense of being in tune with life.

For how could I be otherwise when Change-with-a-capital-C was the only constant that I could see? Why would I friction-burn my mind and fray my heart, trying to hold onto the vagrants of my thinking—a thinking structured by convention into "happy-ever-after"? Happiness ebbs, oscillates. Happiness is tidal.

So, trusting in the process of probabilities, I held onto nothing. I saved neither money nor bottles nor books nor men. Nothing was "mine" but a deep-seated sense of meaning, of the ultimate goodness of things. My curiosity ballooned across the African landscape, led me mostly into "Where am I now? How interesting!" and rarely into "Am I safe? Am I secure?".

I did not want marriage. Or babies. Or to be looked after. From men I wanted company, friendship, humour. Yes, sometimes I wanted their bodies too. With my subsequent lovers, in Africa, France, and back again in England, I enjoyed sexual friendship, which, as the sixties gave way to the seventies, gradually became more acrobatic. And practices hitherto labelled as damnable by my own home-grown Thought-Police, such as oral sex, then smoking-dope-before-sex, and then talking-with-lovers-*about*-sex, were nudged into my picture by an increasingly outrageous Hollywood. But while the movies and the media had begun to tell me that if I was not getting good sex I was not a complete person, I was in fact still more interested in my ardent lovers' *ideas*, in their sense of purpose, in their speculations about why they were on the planet, than I was in their male members.

Not so, however, with Noel. The Canadian who said to me in the summer of 1978, "I think we should get married", and to whom I replied, "Alright, let's do that". And me thirty-four years old.

We met among the broad-bodied, flat-footed mountain people of Papua New Guinea. I was teaching English to the grandchildren of a Stone-Age culture that whiteskins first came upon as recently as 1933. And he? He ran the movie projector Friday nights at the local sports club, a circular grass hut of huge diameter. "Heard you were coming", he boomed without artifice. No literary allusions here. No jests in Latin. Kindness barrelled from him, the sort of kindness and directness that has been composted in the gardens of North American Protestantism, and blossoms disarmingly, fully aware of itself.

Among the New Guinea Highlands men there was little nostalgia lost between the harsh traditional life dominated by the elements and the new entrepreneurial ways of the whiteskins. The petrol stations, the weaving sheds, the coffee plantations that Noel (employed by the Papua New Guinea government) helped them to run, offered them something new: the comforting arms of economic security.

He was popular. He was impressive. He was submerged in the economic mainstream and patently unimpressed by my quoting of Kurt Vonnegut's immortal definition of the American Dream: *Grab too much, or you'll get nothing at all* ...

His unabashed interest in sex, and, what was new for me, his wish to give pleasure as well as take it, led me down as yet uncharted paths of my own sexuality. There were times when, yes, he filled my senses; times when the fire of our meeting burned up our boundaries and we became a force far greater than us both, a channel for achieving the remarkable, a channel for Life to do its work. These were the times when the dry bones of my mother's words — "It's 'orrible" — lay scattered by storms of passion.

There were other times too—when I was sitting over my astrology books and charts; when I was writing; when I was planning a lesson that would make students say "what!" and "really?"; when I was making paradoxical associations in my mind; when we had both dropped acid and laughed ourselves ill at the apparently preposterous sight of the post office building—times when my new lover's invitations to bed or living-room floor were not necessarily accepted.

We were now entering a new era. The sixties had left their legacy of Screaming Sex. It came at us from all corners of the developed world—from the TV, the cinema, the music industry. Protruding, gaping and threatening from the windows of every twopenny-half-penny rickety-rackety newsagent shop run by old ladies in bedroom slippers were tits, bums, chains and whipping-posts.

I looked for meaning in this. Could find it only in money. Rock stars and newsagents have to eat, and the British had foisted the Economic Social Theory upon the world, that altar upon which the genius of humanity, latent within the hearts of those same rock stars and newsagents, has been sacrificed.

When Noel came with me to England to meet the old crowd, we talked of these things, looking out through the unwashed windows of the grim Tilbury-line train. From the City of London to the appropriately-named Grays, the frayed and hopeless landscape could offer no more of itself to society's enduring religion: industrial growth. The familiar sight depressed me. "The only way we know how to live is by robbing the planet, shitting in our own backyards", I said.

"What do you mean?" he asked.

"Look out there", I nodded towards the wasteland. "That's how we rich people, I mean rich in relative terms, maintain our standard of living. By robbing nature."

He looked, finally saying, "I've never thought about it that way before ..."

I knew him as one who genuinely believed that the new religion of development would liberate people from hostile nature. His image of nature was in accordance with that of economic analysis — a competitive image. When we are taught that competition for commodities "makes the world go round", that is how we see the world. That is how he saw the world, coming, as he did, from upper-middle-class Canada, from the most human-centred religion of all, orthodox Christianity. Coming from parents big in the church. Success in the marketplace is the measure of your godliness.

To strengthen my own tenuous hold on what *he* understood as security, he had offered himself. "What will you do?" he had asked as I studied the world map in preparation for the completion of my two-year contract in Papua New Guinea.

"I don't know."

So he had turned his back on wanting to stay there and came with me, to accompany me in my not knowing.

It was short-lived, that time of not being industrious. For a few months we busily lacked respectability in New Zealand, in Australia, in Indonesia. Until I allowed my not knowing to get boxed, packaged in his banking job in the aspiring and breathless city of Toronto, Canada.

Noel thus pursued success in the marketplace while I, cradled in the assurance of his bass voice and the promise of his man's arms, began to beat time with something new, began to beat time with security. I allowed him to collect for both of us, to collect books and bottles and furniture, a house. He looked good and he looked after me, in accordance with Hollywood Principles. That he was seven years my junior seemed not to matter.

I cut capers around freelance editing work, studied astrology, had a book published about my extraordinary students in Papua New Guinea, still hearing the songs of the trees and the stars, though they were far, far away.

In Toronto the winters were frigid enough to crack the bones and the teeth inside me. Much of the money for which we exchanged our time, our lives, was spent upon keeping ourselves insulated against this threat from the very air. I have no Innuit blood. I could not be a friend of this air.

This air, it seemed to me, lent an urgency to the marketplace in which Noel busied himself. Survival in this air required considerable attention. If you hung around a street corner chatting for longer than fifteen minutes you could die of exposure.

The friend I now recalled, vividly and with longing, was warm. Warmth had run through my story since childhood; a golden-green land and the bush singing with changes, with life and with death. These were the gods I had to serve. These were part of my myth.

Oh yes, I can give all sorts of reasons for the things I feel impelled to do, but a "reason" is just a supposedly-logical way of explaining what *really* motivates me. And what *really* motivates me is that sense that *there is something that I ought to be doing ... some purpose to my life ... but I cannot quite remember where I put it.* This mislaid sense of purpose is what the English Buddhist monk, the Venerable Sangharakshita, calls myth.

So my myth brought us back to Australia, which had delighted us both in our three-month journeying down the east coast and then up from Adelaide, through flocks of parrots and ancient mauve-pink dawns, to Darwin. Here I had heard again the whispers of the gods of the land, the whispers I had shared with friends at primary school.

I wanted to head straight for the country. Friends told us about the north coast of New South Wales, but Noel hooked a good job in Sydney. He talked of the necessity of "paying the bills", turned quietly from my argument that the life attendant upon mainstream jobs itself creates the biggest bills.

In 1983, three weeks after the birth of our first and only child, a son, Jack, we came to Sydney. Well if we have to live in a big city, let's *really* live in a big city. I wanted a community—Paddington? Newtown? Redfern? Let's have people in our lives, for our baby's sake if nothing else. Surrogate uncles and aunts for him, surrogate brothers and sisters. I was thirty-nine. Unlikely to have another child. Retaining my distaste for the life of the copulating couple cooped up cosily with kids, I did not want us to be the only adults in our son's life; sensed the lack of wisdom in such a situation, the folly of the nuclear family niche.

Noel wanted us both in "a nice home". I had already compromised him over the move to Australia. It had been hard on him, leaving his family, leaving his job promotion. In addition, I was a spiritual slouch. I had not the will to insist, again, that we jointly follow my heart. It was too hard for me to rail convincingly against the lovely-suburban-house-and-garden-with-space-for-a-swimming-pool. I rather liked it.

For eight years the only cause of our rare arguments was my odd outburst over wanting to live somewhere else and some*how* else. In the country. Where we could see the stars touching the horizon. Where we could become part of a community pursuing myths other than *get as comfortable as you can regardless of the cost to others.*

Living *somehow* else. That is what would bend me into thought at the end of every visit to the super-dooper-market, or whenever Noel came home with unnecessary commodities, visible proof of "buying power". How to live *somehow* else and still not lose my loved ones. I played with organic foods, encouraged Noel along to foster-parent training, admired active alternates from a distance.

Dad came from England, nearly ninety years old, on remarkably purposeful legs, to live with us. We made a grandad flat. We spoiled him, he who had talked to my child's wide eyes about the stars. He too was drawn into their music.

I freelanced in publishing, wrote stories about families and rainforests and meaning, meaning, meaning. I began to notice like-minded people, began to find friends whose eyes met mine. We knew that "freedom" has little to do with the fulfilment of material need, little to do with the conquest of nature. Freedom is a personal path, and as much as people are free in their individual creative expression, that much will they connect with and inspire others. Some of my new friends were of the Western Buddhist Order, a non-monastic order that treads its difficult path along with mortgages and jobs and children. From them I learned the techniques of Buddhist meditation. With them I recalled a poem by Narihira:

*I have always known*
*That at last I would*
*Take this road, but yesterday*
*I did not know that it would be today.*

Occasionally I tugged on the invisible cord I felt connecting my life with the golden-green hills of the north coast of New South Wales. As holidaymakers, Noel and Jack and I had visited the hills at the back of Byron Bay, far far north of Sydney, where there is a community that views economic rationalists as the lunatic fringe. Then, just like that, after eight years in the city, Noel asked the bank for a transfer, and got it. Permission to be paid for working out of Lismore and Ballina, towns that abut those same soft hills.

I did the packing.

We let the house in Sydney.

We bought green hectares studded with dots of rainforest and bounded by a platypus-and-turtle-filled river, from which (if you stand in just the right spot) not one electric light can be seen at night.

Only the stars.

Only the stars.

Under the stars and on our first night there, Dad raised his glass and said to us, "May you prosper all your days".

Two days later he was dead.

I injured my back trying to lift him. I almost ruptured a disc.

❖ ❖ ❖

When I read nearly thirty years ago Kurt Vonnegut's *God Bless You, Mr Rosewater*, I hooted with all the pleasure of recognising a fellow-traveller as Eliot Rosewater crashed a convention of science-fiction writers and addressed the scribes thus:

> *I love you sons of bitches ... You're all I read any more ... You're the only ones zany enough to agonize over time and distances without limit, over mysteries that will never die ...*
>
> *The hell with talented sparrowfarts who write delicately of one small piece of one mere lifetime, when the issues are galaxies, eons, and trillions of souls yet to be born.*

I knew thirty years ago that I was a mythic being, a being essentially outside time and space that had somehow got to fit her purpose inside time and space. But as I experienced it then, time and space was a damper, a spent squib, the prison of burning-your-toast-in-the-mornings, or getting-lit-up-because-somebody-on-the-Underground-smiled-at-you. To hell with the small, the personal. I am large ... I contain multitudes ...

Consequently, like Eliot Rosewater, I too used to read nothing but science-fiction. And, again like Vonnegut's hero, I could be surly about it. The hell with individual lifetimes. The hell with the microcosm.

No more. Now that I am fifty, I see ... what do I see? I see that individual lives are as full of paradox as galaxies, eons, and trillions of souls yet to be born. Paradox in daily life might not be as easy to recognise as it is on the galactic level. Time and space have a way of healing over the paradoxes and ironies that flesh is heir to. And, looking back, we make ourselves believe the version of things that makes most "sense" to us. A version so lacking in the daily absurdity of personal detail as to be meaningless.

Now I see that individuals reflect every other individual, like the pearls in Indrah's Net, the Hindu symbol of universal connectedness. And when, after Noel, Jack and I settled onto our beautiful forty hectares, I felt a kind of lurching inside that heralded not just the change inherent in moving house, but The Change with a big T and a big C. I was forty-seven.

To record the contradictions I felt looming in life, so that I would not as an old lady be tempted to look back on these years and package them in one nice-trite-theory, the sort of easy-peasy extrapolation our society and its newspapers are so fond of, I began this journal in November 1992. I addressed it to Noel, wrote it to him, did not want him, either, to let these years go in confusion or over-simplification.

When I decided to seek publication, I changed some names. And I did a lot of cutting, staying only with my marriage, my menopause, my freedom. There has been much more for me in these years than what finally appears here. My heart has travelled other places of pain and joy. It has wept with the people of Bosnia and Rwanda. It has danced with the dismantlers of apartheid. Invariably though, it has come back here. Because here is where I can act. Here is a place where, finally, I for one and those that may yet live with me, might cease to rob nature.

The astrology I refer to in my journal is the harmonics of the planets — called the transits. As the planets move they form certain angles to the birth-chart's original planetary positions and other sensitive points. The angles, planets and points involved during a transit are symbols for various passages through life.

Centuries of observation by people better equipped to comment than sceptics who know nothing but the pop astrologer's "stars" column, shows the transits for what they probably are. Not fortune-telling pointers, but symbols of our spiritual intent. The transits are part of the "gold in the dung heap of astrology", to use the words of Johan Kepler, the great astronomer who at the turn of the seventeenth century drew up the laws governing the movement of the planets.

Just like my childhood-heart, such as it now is, the time-honoured understanding of astrology does not see the will of human beings in opposition to that of the universe. It is not a question of Us-and-It. It is the Us-and-It notion that has given rise to Evil. To Satan. To the Enemy. The Enemy is a handy thing for the Military-Industrial-Complex to have around. No wonder its scientists, upholders of the hard-and-fast-laws-of-nature, threw astrology out the window.

Like all writing, this journal is just a line of words. The writing is not *me*, the author. It is a line of words that caught at certain moments when I was awake enough to set the snares. Moments come and moments go. Sometimes experienced as sad, sometimes as happy. This line of words has snaked along my moments these past few years, twining itself around this or that standpoint, sometimes leading me and at other times being led.

Like the planets, the wordshapes are symbols too. They are not *the truth*. And in recognising that they are not *the truth* I may be reminded that in this small time I came to understand why the probable and undogmatic universe of quantum physics had always appealed to me. Just like my life, it describes a dance of inter-being.

My love, my marriage, my family have changed with my Change. The few doors left ajar before me do not have large handsome men waiting behind them, ready to sweep me up a plush staircase of social, sexual and economic expectation.

What those doors now open to is the child-wisdom I lost in my storm-tossed years of fertility—a wisdom that told me there are people we can love completely, but without complete understanding.

# The Journal

Of course we'd like to keep the ideal picture we have of ourselves. I'd like to believe that I'm a fine mother: patient, understanding, wise. (If only my children would agree with me, it would be nice!) But still, this nonsense of emotion-thought dominates our lives.

Particularly in romantic love, emotion-thought gets really out of hand. I expect of my partner that he should fulfill my idealized picture of myself. And when he ceases to do that (as he will before long) then I say, "The honeymoon's over. What's wrong with him? He's doing all the things I can't stand." And I wonder why I am so miserable. My partner no longer suits me, he doesn't reflect my dream picture of myself, he doesn't promote my comfort and pleasure. None of that emotional demand has anything to do with love. As the pictures break down—as they always will in a close relationship—such "love" turns into hostility and arguments.

Charlotte Joko Beck
*Everyday Zen*

## Sunday 1 November 1992

Looking at your Herculean back in bed this morning; getting little whispered messages of changes to come; feeling, knowing the menopause will happen in the next year or three; deciding to write to you about it, about the Change, about the changes, so that when we are older, together or apart, we might read these words, share them with our son, and all of us understand a little more ...

Where was I? Bed. This morning. Day twenty-eight of my cycle. Good. Normally it should have started on day twenty-one. Let's hope my customary three-week cycle means my eggs have been depleted that much more quickly and I blossom into menopause before fifty. Felt almost elated at the prospect.

Turned in bed, away from your oblivious back, then imagined I felt the wetness of bleeding. Please, don't let it be. Let's miss this one. Let's start missing them and missing them. The herald of the menopause — missed periods. Yeah! Let's really get stuck into this business of erratic cycles, concrete proof of fertility winding down. I had a feel, then looked at my fingers. Yes! No blood.

Nasty in the back though. For the past week, pain from my disc protrusion and feelings of PMT. All symptomatic. But — no blood.

To the Byron markets today, and I managed to stop paying attention to the back pain. Bought baggy silk pants for self and a kite for Jack. Enjoyed being together, happy at the prospect of being able to tell people "I'm menopausal, you know" because that statement has the ring of authority about it, the ring of crone-like wisdom; and I said to you, "Nah, I don't think this period's going to happen because I feel so good". You looked sceptical, as I notice you often do when you look at me these days. You also looked abundantly healthy.

Well. We got home. I went to the loo. And there was the familiar dark smear on the knickers. Sigh.

## Monday 2 November

I did some gardening this morning and later read Chapter Ten of Germaine Greer's *The Change*. Not the book I was hoping it would be. I wanted to read about *her* experiences, not all those long-forgotten Gallic women, dead for 300 years and more. Anyhow, this chapter, on alternative treatments, had some interest:

> *Alcohol burns off the small post-menopausal oestrogen supply and interferes with calcium metabolism ... Coffee and salt can cause calcium to be secreted ... The best way to approach the climacteric is to be in shape. The menopausal woman should cut down her total food intake ...*

Now I already knew much of this. But I needed to read the words to know I knew it. It's what I've been telling myself for the last year and more. The year of living in the slow and lonely lane, the lane where I've travelled inside myself and found I don't want to do this or that any more. Because I'm changing.

Alcohol will be the hardest. The occasional evening drink still turns into two or three more often than I like. And the superannuated cells of my body, mere shadows of their ancestors of 1960s vintage, gasp out their response not just one day, but two or three days after the fact.

Tea and coffee? No problem. I don't intend cutting out these things completely. Never was a subscriber to the prohibition mentality. Just cut down; be kind to myself, kind but firm. I'll also fast one day a week. On Mondays, when you're away and dinner need only be got for Jack. Twenty-four hours each week without food.

## Tuesday 3 November

I fasted today since I missed out yesterday. And you were away anyway. Fine at first. Lots of mineral water, juice. At 4 p.m. I pick up Jack from school to take him to a riding lesson. Headache starting. OK. Normal. I've fasted before. For *days*. Though it was years ago. First day or two always bad. Will take time for body to adjust to a day a week without food.

Got home and headache raging. Lay down for ten minutes to breathe the monster away, but all to no avail. Then it occurred to me I'd been without food for longer than twenty-four hours anyway, from yesterday's dinner to now. So at 7 p.m. I boiled two eggs for myself, fresh from the chook house, wholesome gifts from my Australorp girls, my feathered racehorses, falling over one another to get to the treats I bear them each day. Delicious, record-size brown eggs. No salt, no pepper. Soft boiled. Headache dissolving before my very eyes.

Onto Jack's spelling list, feeling fine. I'd actually been thinking of doing a longer fast, thirty-six hours, from Sunday evening to Tuesday morning. But no. I won't do that. Slowly, slowly woman. Be kind, be cautious.

The period has been as usual. Not a lot of bleeding. Basically over with now.


## Thursday 5 November

Cleaned the house for Petrov family (friends from Melbourne) arrival. A lot of back pain. Shouldn't be this bad when I'm not pre-menstrual. But there it is.

Later in the day I turned into a werewolf. You had got home from work later than usual. You'd promised to take Jack and me out to dinner with your winnings from the Melbourne Cup. You'd also told Keri you'd take the chainsaw over to her place to cut down a few trees around where she's building. I suggested you phone Keri to put that off till the weekend. No, you said. It wouldn't take long. Only a couple of trees. We'd still get to the restaurant by 7.30. "So you're going over to Keri's?" I said, suddenly angry. "Yes, it won't take long."

I didn't believe that; I started stomping around, making beds as noisily as it's possible to make beds, while you and Jack got organised to go. We'll be late to the restaurant. Jack will be late to bed. School in the morning. Fume. Finally I yelled out the window—yelled, mind you, something I do not do, but I did it now and it felt so good, that surge of adrenalin: "Will you bloody get going!"

Your face aghast, as though I'd shot you in the kneecaps: "What's the matter with *you*!" was your reasonable response.

I was being carried along. Not responsible. "Bloody get going! It's late enough already!" There was more: "And did you measure that space for that log in the vegetable garden!" It wasn't a question. I knew you hadn't.

You confirmed this. "No."

"No," I came back, "I didn't think you would! Because it's for me!"

Even as I was saying this to you, I knew it was complete codswallop. But I reached my objective. I succeeded in making you angry. I stood self-satisfied as you measured the space in the vegetable garden with sudden movements, reported back to me in abrupt tones, got in the car with Jack and burned rubber. Then the skies opened and I was left hoping you'd get stuck in the mud.

Five minutes later when I'd quietened down I didn't have to wonder what that had all been about. Keri. Ten years younger than me. And isn't she lovely looking? You and she share some interests to which I'm indifferent (cattle, beer). I like her. She is a kind person; I appreciate the help she's given us, sharing her knowledge of the countryside around here, her hospitality.

I cried. I was feeling utterly pathetic, having to kneel

down to make the beds because I couldn't bend. You returned easily in time to make the restaurant by 7.30. I apologised. Said my fear was that the back pain and whatever else it was that I was going through would get worse and make me unpleasant to live with, that I'm finding it hard to be good to other people when I'm feeling bad about myself. Jack gave me a cuddle. So did you. Thanks.

## Monday 16 November

How is it possible for me to be thinking I'm "in love" with the physiotherapist? When I've been moving through these last few years secure in my thinning hormones and sedate demeanour and my ability to admire men without reference to their genitalia?

But God, he's beautiful. After my second treatment I was having to tell myself to be reasonable. After my third treatment I was having to tell myself that I *was* being reasonable. Perfectly reasonable. "I don't want to have a relationship with him", my perfectly reasonable mind told me as it left his clinic and weaved itself through the traffic and up into the stratosphere. "Who wants a relationship that could ruin both our marriages? No. I just want to use him for sex."

I'm fantasising between treatments. Monday night I dreamt he kissed me. He's dogging my thoughts and my daily meditation. I'm astounded. My new resolve to be healthier, eat less, look better, has taken on an urgency. I want him to notice me. To think me beautiful and funny and sensitive.

Noel, I don't know if you still find me beautiful and funny and sensitive. Do you? You've said nothing along those lines for some time. And I don't know that even if you did, even if you suddenly came at me with flowers and poetry and praise, I don't know that it would make any difference to this need I feel for the physio to fall wildly in love with me.

And I want him to think me kind, so if he does reciprocate he will know I'm not out to dash his family and ours upon the rocks of mid-life passion. How is this possible? Who knows!

Last Wednesday morning the Petrov family returned to Melbourne. Saw them off on the bus. Picked up the milk from Keri's, then back home to change for my treatment. I chose a close-fitting sleeveless top and the emerald green pants. Looked good. A bottler in fact. Remarkable what clothing can do.

But he didn't get to see the ensemble. I had to take off the top and don something resembling a flour-bag while his assistant gave me a deep-tissue massage. After this he came in. I'm standing there in the flour-bag. Our eyes met. Something made me think he knows, my God he knows I dreamed about kissing him. I smiled more than I should and felt like a bowl of jelly throughout the whole treatment.

We talked. Newtonian physics. Metaphysics. Meditation. Being sensitive to the big picture. All the time his piano-player fingers are upon me. I try to choose my words mindfully. But I ache. Oh, how I ache.

We talked about you. You who gave me his phone number for Jack's slight scoliosis. "Try this bloke", you said, having had your neck fixed by him. And I liked the way he was with Jack, decided to try him myself.

"Is Noel into meditation, that kind of thing?" he asks. Why does he ask? Might he think you don't understand me? I do hope so. But I'm circumspect. I smiled mysteriously and told him you were "getting there", though I'm not sure of the truth of that.

The weekend has come and gone since then. I did a lot of gardening. Thought less about the physiotherapist. I enjoyed planting the two Illawarra flame trees with you. In the paddock in front of the house. But I did *not* enjoy that later conversation when you (again) broached my reluctance to "generate income" over the last year or so. Again we talked across the ideological chasm between us. On my side there is enough "material" for one small family and on your side there is always room for more, just in case. Told you again how I'd grown to dislike the dogsbody work I'd been doing in publishing for years, albeit as a freelancer; how I now need to be more creative in what I do, more self-expressive; how finding that self-expression will take time; how I believe I'm menopausal and sensing many changes, and that Change with a capital C is on its way and I will not remain in these hormonal doldrums for ever.

Told you all that. But you weren't impressed, were you?

## Tuesday 17 November

I don't consider I need any further affirmations of the fact that there's a "nugget of gold in the dung heap of astrology", as Johan Kepler himself described it. BUT, my oath, here is a thing. Following further dreaming upon the divine physiotherapist, I looked at my planetary transits chart last night, as I do from time to time. It's often these retrospectives that give me the nicest thrill when it comes to validating what science chose to dismiss. No chance of a self-fulfilling prophecy here.

*Et voila.* What do I find? Pluto is squaring my natal Venus. Exact now and remaining within orb through the whole of next year. Exact NOW. Astrologer extraordinaire Robert Hand, in his book *Planets in Transit*, says "relationships may become a source of challenge" under this transit. Yes. How interesting. But wait—there's more. There's talk of an urgent desire for love, of a possibility of grabbing whoever is available instead of waiting for someone who might be better suited. Talk of becoming so besotted by this person that you do not see them as they really are. Robert Hand goes on to tell me that even if I am happily married I could become strongly attracted to someone else — and this could "disrupt" my marriage.

Well now. Here comes the *really* interesting bit. Because I am experiencing certain drives that are not operating in accordance with my best interests, I am advised to cool it, to distance myself from involvement with my current sex-god and wait out the situation. See what happens when the dust has settled, the flames have died down. And it is possible, says the oracle, that something beneficial and abiding will arise from my considered approach to the passion.

Furthermore, Pluto squaring Venus may point up all sorts of problems that have existed for who-knows-how-long in the marriage relationship. Either partner may display jealousy and a reluctance to allow the other freedom to be who they are. I think both Noel and I are guilty of that. But I more so. Hand stresses the importance of honest communication at this time; that this transit brings with it an opportunity for profound change in the relationship. "A bad one may end," he writes, "but a good one will become deeper."

Two thoughts ran parallel through my mind when I read what he had to say: firstly, what does he mean by advising against giving into temptation, and secondly, is there any way round that, I wonder — is it possible to pull a fast one on the cosmos? And two, what price the old saying "The heavens do not impel, they incline", when they're clearly inclining *me* to an impelling degree?

I've been struck many times before by the appropriateness of the planetary symbolism at certain turns in my life. This is another such time.

## Sunday 22 November

The solitude is delicious. Even though it was mostly by my organisation that we had twenty people here last night for a "pot luck" dinner, I didn't really want to talk to any of them. Though I think I was gracious enough.

Today I am all alone. You are away for two days — seminar and work. Jack spending the weekend with a friend.

This morning I meditated. Lay in the sun. Showered. Concerned solely with my own thoughts. It feels indulgent. It is indulgent. There is some sadness around the edges at the apparent lack of direction in my life just now. But it's tempered by a canny sort of surety that outside this ball I now find myself curled up in — sometimes with the blankets literally over my head — is a sense of purpose and an opportunity for fulfillment greater than anything I've experienced before.

Keeping house, husband and son has been and still is a part of this metamorphosis, but it seems to me that the well-being that defines the heart of me will one day have carried me beyond the housekeeper and the wife; beyond what I see as, basically, an economic relationship; and into — who knows? A relationship based on something less self-serving, like love. And the mother? I don't know. Can one ever stop being a mother?

I've no idea where the passionate feelings for the physiotherapist fit into this cosmic picture. I'm not trying to analyse; only observe. Writing about it helps the observation, helps put some distance between myself and the emotion; the same purpose that is served by meditation.

I had another treatment last Wednesday. On my way to the clinic, I bumped into someone I knew. "You look great", she said, "your face is sparkling". Ah, the narcotic of thinking you're in love. It has wrought the miracle of a sparkling 48-year-old face and less back pain too.

*He* told me I looked good too. We spent the first ten minutes talking about our respective experiences of meditation and profundity. My heart was audible, palpable through the saggy daggy flour-bag. "Good to meet a serious meditation practitioner", he said as treatment started. Ooh, yes. Boom boom. I told him about the little meditation hut down by the river, that I go down there for my sit each morning around 5.30. "Does Noel mind?" he enquired. Why? I wonder why. I told him how you helped build the hut. "Noel knows that my meditation practice is important to me, gives me support."

"My wife is a Born Again Christian", he said. My heart sank for him and leapt for me.

"Oh."

"That's alright", he added, "I can deal with that ... Do you know about the Born Agains?" Why was he telling me all this?

"I've talked to a few and I've heard the song 'I'll See You in the Rapture'. I like talking to Christians who like theology. I'm interested in the Saviour idea, the needing something external, deferring to something external, the 'putting your faith in ...', like the Catholic Indulgences of old: put the money in the box and it'll be all better. It seems to me a rejection of serious self-observation."

I was trying to be rational and objective when all the while my mind was racing with thoughts of how much better this was going than I had imagined in my moments of catatonic staring at the ceiling. He was nodding furiously at everything I was saying. He loves me, he loves me. He's flirting with me. Or ... is he *really* interested in what I'm saying?

For the first few days after this I felt all the positive

aspects of being in love colouring my surroundings. It enhanced my communication with you. I felt happier in myself and with myself than I had in an age. I noticed how much more patient and pleasant I was with you. I gave long deep thought to how, if I were to have a discreet affair with the physio, which I don't want to do and I do want to do, it would have no bearing on my love for you. You are Noel, separate from the physiotherapist. You are a part of me, a part of my story. To reject you would break my heart, break Jack's heart. Must affairs necessarily do that?

I have heard "philandering" males use this argument — that their affairs don't change their love for their wives. I don't know if I could myself use such an argument and continue to maintain that my life is that of spiritual seeker. I don't *know* if I could. But I feel forced into thinking about it ...

## Monday 23 November

Much of this morning's meditation taken up with thoughts I couldn't distance myself from. I am confronted by conclusions I reached years ago, indeed was probably *born with*, given my vivid memory of asking my primary school friends why on earth they should want so much to get married.

I was talking to you in my mind, Noel, on my way back to the house after meditation. This is what I was saying: "Why should we, knowing and liking and loving one another as we do, loving our child as we do, and wishing to remain together for those reasons, why should we be sexually jealous of one another?" Why not permit one another the happiness and fulfillment another sexual relationship might bring?

I've been jealous. Witness the recent outburst over Keri.

What was it? All of three weeks ago? Now, in the light of my passion for the physio I'm thinking that if you would like another woman I'd be quite obliging. Let's give one another a free hand on this issue.

To be fair to myself, I *have* said as much to you before —remember? I have said to you that if you wanted "an affair", I wouldn't necessarily go berserk and want to break up the family over it. It would depend on the dynamics of the situation. Obviously I wouldn't want to hear all the details, but at the same time I would not want to be deceived. I would not want to be lied to. I think of wives who are lied to for years on end and I am appalled for them. I cringe at the lack of respect, trust, decency and love. I have told you that if you were discreet and honest with your "other" woman, and if she made you feel happier (for you are not a happy person, not in the way I am, you take no pleasure in little things), then you may even have my blessing. I have told you this.

But I've never asked you if you would reciprocate such largesse! I fear not. I can't be certain, but I think an affair on my part would lead to acrimony and breakup.

In the past, as I understand it, sex did not have so much to do with defining marriage. It was not the sex that bonded a couple, as is the case nowadays. Marriage was a question of survival; still is, in some parts of the world, mostly the poor parts. In those so-called underdeveloped countries where I spent so many years, where life was lived according to older traditions, the children grew up with many more than two adults for their role models. Their lives were filled with aunts, uncles, grandparents and many others. Kids were almost public property, liable to score cuddles or praise or a cuffed ear from any one of a number of carers. So it was no great thing if their biological parents did not "have a relationship" in the sanctified sense we imply when we use that term.

Jack has no family apart from us. My English family

are either dead or busy and your Canadians are a long, long way away. I will not sour his childhood by raising the spectre of separating parents.

This is my harvest. Marry late in life. Have babies late in life. Still have the responsibility of them as children when menopause whispers in your ear its messages of solitude/freedom/and-men-that-might-suit-you-more.

## Tuesday 1 December

I'm not reading my previous entries. That way this journal will be truly ephemeral. I don't wish to consider what I've already written. One day I'll sit down and read the complete document. Could be an insight into what Buddhism calls Impermanence. Or could be a good laugh. Or perhaps both.

Indolence. I've never been so indolent. Oh I'm doing things, perhaps quite a lot compared with some people. A little teaching. Some writing. Gardening. Planting trees. But still I feel indolent, and needing to sleep a lot. Eight to nine hours each day, counting the afternoon lie-down that became necessary with the back injury. But I used to be a six-hour-maximum-type sleeper. I used to have boundless energy when I barely knew what to do with it. Now I have a vision of turning the cattle paddocks into the Fields of Elysium and I can't even start the lawn mower.

I tell myself this time will pass. And of course it will. It's a rite of passage. Let us sit back, or stay with head under the bedclothes, and see what happens.

## Thursday 31 December

What now? It's a while since I wrote. Lack of inclination. Mindless, lazy Christmas with just the three of us, for the first time in years. And Chittaprabha ("Radiant Mind") — dearest friend, meditation teacher, mentor. She, who when I first met her and before I knew she was a musical-scientist-Buddhist-grandmother had me thinking, "Here is a person I will be friends with, who knows things that I want to know too". Chittaprabha, here from Sydney for a whole week till Christmas Eve! Sitting together, swimming together, shopping in Woolies. There was a sense of normalcy in having her here. We share that sense — quiet joy at the pleasurable times and equanimity in the face of the ghastly. All quite normal. Yet I could, and sometimes do, write poems about it.

It's New Year's Eve now and she's gone. You and Jack lit a fire in the brazier outside. Half moon. Jupiter virtually lighting up the surrounding sky. Brilliant night. Jack and friend Ben all knees and elbows toasting marshmallows and racing round with sparklers. I played music. You oversaw it all till 10 o'clock, when you could no longer stay awake. You and the boys were all asleep by 10.30. But I felt like writing.

Ah my stir-fry. Every vegetable in tonight's dinner, bar the onion, was from my garden. The authenticity of it! Offering plates full of your own produce to family and friends is a blow struck for freedom from economic tyranny. Decrepit I may be, but as I bend my back painfully to harvest my shallots, I am in step with the great dance of life!

## Monday 11 January 1993

I am still not looking back on these entries. Let them reflect the Indrah's Net of my mind. Let them reflect the divine Walt Whitman:

> *Do I contradict myself?*
> *Very well then, I contradict myself.*

*I am large, I contain multitudes.*

Whatever I was saying about the physiotherapist ... it's all changed. I am no longer "in love". At his suggestion I went to a public talk on health and nutrition while a friend from England was staying with us and I could ill afford the time. I went to gaze upon his long lean frame and fantasise that he was mad for me. But his wife was with him, a small quiet person who clung at his side all night. How could he have brought *her* along? Didn't he know, didn't the very Ether of Creation let him know we had a date? And me looking as good as I did! I began to detach on sight of her. By the end of the evening, when he came to sit beside me, the usual penetrating look, the hand gently on my knee and the "Give me a call if you want to follow up the programme ... ", the detachment was complete. It was late. Everyone was tired. At my next treatment he made complimentary sounds about my "lovely olive skin". But I was unimpressed.

Now I know that conditioned existence is subject to change, but at forty-eight years old I'd got used to my emotional base having a bit more stability than that! A few short days before and I would have been squeezing my legs together in joy at such bold overtures as "lovely olive skin". But now I just smiled, and asked about my condition, as any clear-minded patient might.

What was it Robert Hand said in *Planets in Transit*? Avoid the temptation. Such a relationship is basically unstable ... With the cosmos in mind I left his clinic happily and went to do some shopping with Jack.

## Monday 18 January

I am in and out of understanding. After days of feeling I shared my life with a stranger, suddenly I am with a friend. You are galaxies away from me, yet our closeness cannot be denied. We worked together long hours in the garden and paddocks this weekend. Jack helped here and there and was a delight. I have wondered many times if it is only our son that keeps us together. But this weekend I saw it was more complex than that.

I *can* talk to you. This is precious. Sometimes you're an oaf. But I can talk to you about thinking you're an oaf. This is very precious. "He's a hypocrite", said Jack the other day. I was alarmed. Didn't even know the child knew that word, that damning word, that worst of all words. "What do you mean?" I asked.

"He's always going on about saying thank you and having perfect table manners, but *he* hardly ever says thank you and he drinks out of bottles that other people have to use ..."

It was true, my oath.

Sitting with you later, I told you. Not accusations. Just "This is how Jack is reacting. D'you think he's justified?" You listened, agreed that you do sometimes expect too much of Jack and don't always set the example yourself. I was heartened. It was a thoughtful response, though to be fair to you it was not out of character. You're not a particularly defensive person, when one takes the trouble to sit you down, make the eye contact, and lay bare the mind.

Jack has had friends here all holiday. Now he and I are having a few days alone together. I like that. He makes me laugh, though his imaginary worlds are far from those of my girlhood. Where was his mind yesterday, I wonder, when we had quietly arrived home in the car and he immediately flung open the door on his side, leapt out with imaginary weapon held at the shoulder storm-trooper fashion, and yelled into the trees, "THIS MEANS WAR!".

My health is on an even keel. I'm now taking a multi-vitamin tablet and evening primrose oil daily. The general cleaning up of diet, the day's fast each week, the cut-down on alcohol and caffeine, swimming, gardening, walking— all helping, I'm sure.

Occasional pain in the knees and backs of legs. Most often when pre-menstrual. Fortunately mild. Generally my energy is still low. Not uncommon in my female peers. The back pain persists. The physiotherapy helped (leaving aside all reference to my heart). But it's time that's needed. Time, exercise, good food, rest and an awakened compassionate mind in balance with a mind at peace. There, a recipe for fulfillment in decrepitude.

In the night I had that feeling of movement within and the muffled sexual urging that usually precedes my period by ten or so days. When will it end? I must stop asking. I talked to Janice, who at fifty-three still finds herself bleeding occasionally—but only when she's having a sexual relationship—"as though my body's saying: Look! Look! Look! We can still make a little human being!", she joked. Is the reproductive urge that great?

## Thursday 21 January

A few weeks ago I wrote to Chittaprabha that I had begun to admit to myself and others that I no longer had any interest in presenting myself to the world as a professional person, someone "in publishing". All I wanted to do, I wrote, was garden, plant trees, do some personal writing, and love my family. I told her that although I was experiencing this time as a "low", I also knew it would pass; it seemed a quiet preparation for a coming time of achievement in my life. The passion for the physiotherapist swooped in and out of this calm like a tidal wave. It was a "high". What purpose it served I can't say. I suspect it had something to do with clarifying to what extent I'm still, at age forty-eight, a stranger to myself.

Having articulated all this, it was with no small interest that I fell upon another astrological retrospective this very day. I pulled out Marc Robertson's book on the Saturn cycle, *Critical Ages in Adult Life*, a book I've not looked at in years and barely read anyway when I first bought it some fifteen years ago. Saturn's current relationship to my personal chart, according to Robertson, tells me:

*It is time to define the boundaries of your operations ... to lay the foundations of a new round of expression of yourself ... to lay "the anchor" you will always be able to come back to ... Secure "the place you stand personally" — in material, emotional, mental and spiritual terms. And you can do this best by deciding what activities you will move outward into the world from.*

I turned to the oracular *Planets in Transit* for the word on Saturn opposing my Midheaven, and was told that this was a time to "pay very close attention" to my actions, my plans, because I am on the threshold of a new period in my life, a turning point. The time just before this transit often proves very difficult for some people. They feel they are going nowhere, they seem to drift. Yes. As I have noted already in this journal I have felt directionless, and have occasionally thought of my acceptance of this as an indulgence. But no. Why be so WASPish about it?

Robert Hand calls it a "period of preparation". It is the end of a relatively bleak period, from which I shall emerge renewed, gradually moving towards a time of greater fulfillment. Greater outward activity in the world, peaking in fourteen years time, when Saturn comes into conjunction with my Midheaven.

I have a sense of this, without Robert Hand's book. I have told you many times, Noel, that I felt my life would change, would reach fulfillment. That one day it would be *me* that looks after *you*.

And here now I am advised by the great astrologer to put aside "professional" concerns and pay attention to the personal, the domestic.

That is where, at the moment, my greatest responsibility lies.

After reading this, I look at my ephemeris, my tables of planetary movements for the whole of this century. And I saw that the last time Saturn opposed my Midheaven was twenty-eight years ago, second and third years of university, failing my favourite subjects miserably, flitting from one definition of myself to another, directionless, discovering vodka and orange and the insides of toilet bowls.

Following that was my fourteen-year Saturn "upswing" and going "out into the world". And how. Teaching and writing in Africa, Paris, London. Then you find me, Noel, in a tropical paradise at the height of my self-expression, esteem, and professional achievement. Saturn *conjunct* my Midheaven. "You get the job", you said, tossing my published books aside after a cursory glance and then drawing me close. Oh you bottler. You big bearded bottler!

And then, after a few years comes the fourteen-year Saturn "downswing". I turn increasingly inward. I earn less and less, but I am still the only muse you have in your world of economic rationalism. You look after me more and more. You buy us houses. Canada. Australia. You have us comfortable. You joke occasionally about my Pisces Dreaming. The land still runs through my myth. Not cities; not Toronto, London, Paris, Sydney, but land and trees and stars.

Then my baby. Our baby. Quieter still and further inward. "I want to be with the baby. That's my place." My commitment to Buddhism, meditation. Quieter again. And from that still point I tell you at times, "I'll look after *you* one day. I will".

To discover just today, 21 January 1993, the correlation of the Saturn cycle to my life, seems to put me in a pathetic light as a student of astrology. In those early days, nearly twenty years ago, I did nothing but character analyses through natal charts. Bah! It is in the planetary transits that Kepler's golden nugget of astrology can be found.

Later, I spread the charts and readings before you; you who ask me regularly what's going on with your own transits — and always at significant times for you, as we both know.

Thought it was time to share my myth with you. Carried it for years I have, through the grime of all those cities, through the fumes and on the London Underground, the Paris Metro, the Toronto Whatever. Told you I thought we were blessed, that we found ourselves on this beautiful land for a reason. That we could turn it into a rainforest paradise for people to find quiet and contentment. Let the community we live in benefit from it. Don't hold it all close to ourselves alone. Don't think of it as an investment. Let the people and the trees and the river come together.

Told you I'd been thinking about how we should build a meditation sala down by the river where we are re-foresting; about turning the barn into accommodation so fellow-Buddhists could come here to sit amid the birds and the beauty.

Noel, these could be the activities from which I will move outward into the world. Noel? I *never* wanted to be in the mainstream. But I dived into it with you because you were so reliable. And I let you build houses around me because they were so safe. Do you remember that favourite poem of mine by Edna St Vincent Millay? I've quoted it at you often:

*Safe upon the solid rock the ugly houses stand*
*Come and see my shining castle built upon the sand!*

You smile, you smile. Is it wearily? I think it is.
   Pisces Dreaming?
   Let's leave it for today.

## Thursday 11 March

Today I am forty-nine.
   The hiatus continues. A sense of nothing happening.
Even though:
   I've two articles on the go
   My creative writing students praise my teaching
   Our "street" party last week was a great success
   I enjoyed the menopause workshop I attended recently
   And so on ...
   Well. I suppose it's all quite normal. At the workshop
my peers generally agreed that they were experiencing a
sense of hanging in the gap. Said that whether you get the
well-publicised negative symptoms or not, you still know
in your heart that menopause is happening, because you
*feel* so different, so aware of major psychological/spiritual/
life change. The retreating into oneself. The need for
solitude. For reflection upon one's values. Have I upheld
them? Or have I spent my life bouncing off other authorities?
   These were the points we agreed. Though for me it's
impossible to disentangle the menopausal and the atrological
and the this and the that. I know something about the
complex network of reality. For example, that it's a complex
network. But these are the points we all agreed upon.
   I wish you'd been with me. It's clear you don't understand.
How could you? In any sensible social system the women
would be separate from the men at this stage of life. And
really I want very little to do with you. I love and respect
you as a good and kind human being, but I have nil interest
in you as a husband.
   I don't *need* you.
   And you? Do you need me? You who fall asleep in your

armchair, literally, when I talk excitedly about my thoughts, about my "coming of age".

I've no interest in sex with you. It's gone. Dead as a doornail. Bereft of life it rests in peace. Penetration? Ugh! Though I like to cuddle. I like the warmth and love inherent in cuddling. This despite the danger that Germaine Greer warns us of — the numerous fifty-year-old women liking to cuddle and ending up being fucked.

I toy with unilateral declarations of independence; moving into the spare room. But it would hurt you. I can't do that. Why can't I? Why can't I be honest?

I know why. It's Jack. I sometimes think if it were not for our son I would have gone my own way long ago. Perhaps not permanently, but certainly a trial run.

But here we are. Still together in marriage. And quite uncomprehending of one another in key areas of life. Life, Noel, life. Which I don't see as being about economics. I see that *survival* is about economics. Don't you realise how *easy* survival is for people with a half a brain living in this Garden of Eden?

No. Of course you don't. You've been harping more and more on my increasing lack of interest in generating income over this last year or so. I've told you it will pass, this phase, that I'm preparing to open new doors, doors not clearly defined — yet. You don't seem to believe me. No faith in my knowledge of myself, in my prescience.

Well, tough. You're just going to have to put up with it as best you can. I've taken worthless boring work too often in the past for the sake of what you call "paying the bills", when you have always earned enough money to keep us in relative comfort. In a job you say you enjoy, and indeed seem to enjoy.

I think you feel used. I've broached this with you before, but we never seem to get anywhere. I must be more insistent with you. Get you to define yourself to yourself.

But men are bad at that. Fools! You just crash through life, then die.

If you *really* enjoy your work, there is no reason for you to feel used. I suspect you don't enjoy it as much as you say. You're still dripping from the Protestant work ethic you were steeped in as a babe. Sell the house in Sydney. Pay out the mortgage on this place. Throw in your job. You might be a happier person. Start noticing the little things. Like those I do regularly around this too-large home, gardens and paddocks. You might think of putting a flower in a vase for me to find on an unremarked birthday morning. You might say thanks once in a while.

Oh pooh, I don't want to write any more.

## Sunday 14 March

Well now. Look at that last entry. And this morning what did we do? We made love. Nice, it was. And my idea, it was.

There is a moral in this ephemeral material. Me, move into the spare room to keep away from you? Beware, woman, a person does not forget what is said to them in anger or frustration, and the angry and frustrated me is not the whole story. It's not even me. Because there is no "me", as the Zen Master said to the novice. The novice asked the master for help because he was an angry person. "Where is your anger now?" asked the Master, "I want you to show it to me." The student said, "I can't, I'm not angry any more". And the Master concluded, "Well then, obviously it's not you, since sometimes it's not even there".

The moral is tied in with the daily contradictions. Give me depth to accommodate them. Give me wisdom.

You're a reasonable man, Noel. Let's talk, eh?

## Tuesday 20 April

Last day of Jack's Easter school holiday. We made candles. He made a monster twelve-wick single candle, topping yesterday's wick record by a whopping seven wicks. These many-wicked veritable fireworks are his own copyright. The boy's clearly a creative genius. The candle was multi-coloured, but mostly bright green. I was just thinking how like a living organism it looked when Jack, holding it inches above his face and struggling with it in a stranglehold position, croaked up to it, "One step closer and you're doomed!"

The Easter meditation retreat that I organised at the Bodhi Farm went well. Chittaprabha led it with her customary inspiration.

## Wednesday 21 April

I slept a lot yesterday, felt extra lethargic, then discovered why. My period started, about a week early. Very little pain, though a bit headachy. Not enough to stop me from fertilising the 100 trees that you and I planted over the weekend. To each one I had said silently, as I put it in the ground, "To the Earth from the Earth for the Earth".

But I must write now about your news. No more avoiding the issue. You faced me fair and square and told me you wanted Change. Not change, but Change. You didn't go to the demolition derby while I was off on retreat. You had your own "mini-retreat" as you put it, spending virtually the whole week alone. Thinking about us. And you finally acknowledged the tension between us that has been so evident to me for the past year or two and which you have always brushed aside whenever I mentioned it, or else reacted emotionally with, "Why don't you leave if you don't like it?" You said you had reached a point now of being able to look at the tension quite calmly and analytically.

And you felt it had a lot to do with my increasing emotional self-sufficiency, which in turn had to do with my deepening meditation practice and commitment to the Buddhist path. "You don't need people any more, in the sense of clinging to them to bolster your own identity. And I think that's fantastic. I think what's happening to you is fantastic. I'm not blaming anyone or anything for the fact that our paths are diverging. I almost envy you. You don't need to bounce off other people. What power!"

I'd never heard you talk like this before. It was a bit scary. Like having someone you've known for years turn into somebody else.

What's he leading to, I kept thinking, instead of living up to your unwarranted envy and being terribly Zen. Was it a declaration of intent? Was it goodbye?

I told you it wasn't just my meditation, my Buddhism. It was also my age — my menopausal excitement over how much more I can offer life and it can offer me.

Then you fell into a cliché. You said you were tired of being "Mr Nice Guy". Tired and bored with your work. Resentful that I'm off meditating and planting trees and "not getting down to anything mundane". You'd thought about "pissing off" to Bali or Thailand. While you were brushcutting the weeds so that I could plant my trees you were saying, "I don't want to do this. I'm only doing it for her. But she doesn't need or care about me any more".

We talked about sex: my lack of interest in it, your need for it. "I need that warmth, that love. Not just the mechanical thing — may as well just wank. I need that warmth from a woman." Was that the main issue? You said maybe. You didn't know. We talked about my being older than you. Yes, we agreed, it could be that. Could be any number of things ...

I had visions of us building our forest meditation retreat together, organising retreats for people in the community, even catering for them together — we could make our lives here into something honourable; expressions of kindness to people seeking respite from the captains of industry, seeking to deepen their knowledge of themselves and so temper more wisely their responses to others.

This, or something very like it, is to be the expression of my character, which is now of the utmost concern to me. It is no longer a question of having fun. It is a question of knowing that I live my life honourably and with kindness.

Have I become obsessed with this? Have I excluded you, my darling, to such an extent? You whose happiness is so important to me? Before the retreat you asked me how I would define the word "love". I said that to me, loving someone meant that their happiness was just as important as one's own. It didn't mean clinging to them or wanting to keep company with them at all times. It meant what the Buddhists call "mudita"—joy in their joy. You said you thought that was the best definition you had come across. So I knew before the retreat that you were thinking about these things.

And now, after your mini-retreat, you tell me that by my own definition you have loved me all through our marriage. You have put my interests before your own. I know the truth of this. I also know that since we have been married I have ridden on your worldly coat-tails. You have fed, sheltered and clothed me while I have got to know myself. I have shed much of my own conditioning while your middle-class conditioning has kept the flesh on my bones.

Is it now time for the turnaround? Will I now support you as your time comes to turn inward? You asked me a lot of questions about meditation and Buddhism. "Would you like me to teach you to meditate? It may help", I said.

You shrugged. "Maybe sometime."

You said you weren't ready yet. Weren't ready, either, for the forest retreat or my vision of our future together.

"What do you want?" I asked.

You laughed. You said, "Sex and drugs and rock 'n' roll".

I laughed too. Was I remarkable for laughing? When I love you so much? No. But I spit upon the idea of marriage-for-all, just as I spat upon it as a girlchild. And I like honesty, even though it can be painful. We need to face the pain, don't we? Acknowledge it in all its aspects. How else can we then pass on from it, leave it behind, see the new doors opening before us?

"Maybe it's the age thing", you added. Softening the blow? "I'm just not ready for your vision."

You pointed out that in a recent interview I had said to the interviewer that maybe in my dotage I would go to Burma for a while, had a hankering to do so. "You hadn't mentioned that to me at all", you said, "and when I read it I thought where does that leave me? Where do I come in?" This, I suppose more than anything else you had said, made me realise the extent to which I had taken you for granted — my steadfast supporter who no longer feels loved. And yet I love you more profoundly now than I have ever done. How ironic. When we were "in love" it was fun. Fun ruled. Now that I love you, it's not fun at all. You are part of me. Your suffering is mine.

You talked about splitting up, in a theoretical way at first. Then I saw how deeply you had thought about it when you came close to tears as you talked of Jack, of your being incapable of consciously doing anything that would hurt him.

You talked about how your health was suffering. An x-ray had shown some arthritis. You talked about losing your enjoyment of life. About losing your enjoyment of my company.

The following morning, last Friday, we talked more before getting out of bed. Suddenly, and for only a little while, I cried and cried while you hugged me. Then it was over. It was fine. That evening you came home with a gift for me — Sogyal Rinpoche's *The Tibetan Book of Living and Dying*. And you've been reading it yourself ever since, almost unable to put it down, except to help me plant the trees on Saturday.

I think it was sometime on the weekend when we fell to serious talking again that I said to you, "If you do feel the need to get away — to Thailand or wherever — I think you should. You could take a few weeks off work and see how it goes. And if you do find you want sex and drugs and rock 'n' roll, and you intend to come back, please use condoms." At which you laughed. And we reminisced over Graham Chapman's immortal "Give me a packet of French Ticklers, please, for I am a Protestant" in the Monty Python film, *The Meaning of Life*.

## Tuesday 27 April

So you read two passages aloud to me, from my astrology books, describing those current-cosmic-correlations you thought were especially relevant right now in your bewildered life. The first was from *Planets in Transit*, Robert Hand's analysis of Saturn squaring your natal Sun/Mars conjunction. You agreed with everything he said. Yes, you *do* feel discouraged, lacking in energy, challenged on all sides, especially by your employers. You *do* feel people are trying to block you; block your plans, put obstacles in front of you which ever way you turn. Yes, your health *is* suffering as a result of these ego conflicts. Clearly, you were impressed by my "lunatic-fringe" book. But what you found most appropriate of all at this time was a passage from the Marc Robertson book, regarding the Saturn cycle at age forty-one:

> *Personal doubts set in about what* [the individual] *has been doing. He wonders if it has all been worth*

*anything ... The worst manifestation is a kind of noisy*
*confusion about the individual's own worth. Why am I doing*
*all these things? What in the world has it been for? Where*
*have I gone wrong? Questions like that, virtually screamed*
*out to the surroundings, indicate that when the age of 42 to*
*43 arrives, the individual may be in even more*
*confusion ... This is a critical state of psychological*
*adjustment.*

*... [For the "typical cultural type" it is] the beginning*
*of the failing of his physical and emotional vitality. For the*
*creative type, it is not that in any way. In fact, it is one of*
*the peaks of instinctive productive power before one consciously*
*uses that power in the late 40s ... This is a sad period for*
*most individuals who have built their lives around sexual*
*and cultural activities. The "menopause" for both men and*
*women sets in. And if they have nothing beyond their personal*
*attractiveness to lead them beyond this point, the rude*
*awakening begins to set in.*

Well. We both nodded sagely, didn't we? And you've since
dipped into other of my astrology books. In fact you're
showing a healthy interest in holism.

We have covered a lot of ground in this past week. Most
of it on the logistics of giving one another more freedom
from one another while remaining friends, and perhaps
... perhaps ... lovers. You're racing ahead of me though,
in some ways. I'm exhilarated. I'm scared stiff. Part of me
says, "Of course, this *is* what you need to take your life
that step further". Another part of me feels like last year's
calendar tossed in the bin.

You brought up the issue of selling off part of our land
to people committed to reforestation and/or nurturing the
land. What was new in your conversation was that you,
who have always said you would like a house atop this
particular hill, are now bringing this into the picture as
your own separate residence.

And you voiced my daydream, you wily dog ... you said the big house we're living in now would "make a good meditation retreat centre" ... I could live in it, write, teach, organise meditation retreats and other events and oh bliss, bliss, bliss ...

"Could I still sleep with you from time to time, up on the hill?" I asked you. Why did I ask you that? Was it geriatric coquettishness? Or just nostalgia?

Nothing nostalgic about you though, is there? Oh how I envy your lack of sentimentality. "Of course", you said. "But you might have to be prepared to share me with somebody else."

How jealous would I be? Perhaps not at all. Perhaps I should feel wonderfully liberated from having to be "the wife" in every way. Freer to pursue my own ends. No longer thinking of you in terms of a male authority figure, which sometimes I do, but more as a friend. Perhaps even a greater friend, exercising a deeper friendship, than is at present the case.

And how marvellous it could be for Jack, to see us still happy in one another, leading more separate lives yet both more fulfilled. Winding down our conventional marriage as friends. Living close to one another, a walk away. Jack spending time with us separately and time with us together, as circumstances arise. Yes, it could be fine.

And yet what scope for problems, for acrimony. What if your new as yet theoretical woman is painful to me? What if she is idealogically unsound, someone I don't want my son to be around? What if, even if I like her, she becomes possessive of you, resenting time you spend with Jack and me? What if you both fall so wildly in love that we become completely excluded? What if, what if, what if ... how do I know? No point in making up stories and then tracing them over our lives.

The theory is sound. I'll say that again: the *theory* is sound. But I look in the mirror this morning and I see a greying, wrinkling woman, a woman adrift. And suddenly I'm swamped by self-pity. I watch the tears form, let them go. I feel afraid, empty ... and alone. I am suspended over the chasm of middle-age and the options of which way I turn seem pitifully limited. The final choice so much more crucial than the whimsical decisions of my youth.

You are a fine man, Noel. You are yourself undergoing great change. And I know that you are offering me all that is in your heart. I should be grateful, but today I feel only this sadness.

## Thursday 29 April

The last period took me by surprise because it wasn't heralded by the usual increased back pain. I was almost pain-free throughout the meditation retreat, and not once did I have to meditate lying down (which I've had to do at some point in all retreats since the injury). When I got home I felt that the usual back pain would return with the reduction in time spent in meditation. But it didn't. And it hasn't. I've had nothing like the discomfort I was feeling prior to the retreat. And that last period, although it involved heavier bleeding than usual, wasn't marked by any particular discomfort. Though I slept a lot on days one and two. I felt glad to have the opportunity.

There have been some lapses in my food, drink and exercise regimen in the last few months. I've skipped my day of fasting here and there, on the flimsiest of excuses; there have been two or three days when the alcohol consumption has been in the chip-off-the-old-block vein, only to be regretted the following day; and I've gone for as long as a week now and then without thinking about my back-strengthening exercises.

However, today I fasted, to make up for last Monday (when you were home on holidays for Anzac Day), and the Monday before (Easter holidays), and the Monday before (on retreat), and probably the Monday before that too. And I shall fast again next Monday and hopefully for many Mondays thereafter.

I have begun to scout around for more work; I must make an effort at earning more. You become increasingly worried about losing your job — not that it's something you talk about a lot, but I know the concern runs deep. I would prefer to spend time at my own writing. Time with the land. But the Economic Social Theory makes my menopausal longings an indulgence.

Who invented it? The British of course. Adam Smith and his pernicious book *The Wealth of Nations*. Guaranteed to sow the seeds of greed and exploitation. But there it is.

## Friday 30 April

You and I got outside early and planted another thirty-odd trees before the normal workday began. It started out looking as though we were to have another of those stiff-neck, stiff-back, not-meeting-one-another's-eyes differences of opinion that have been so common this last year or two. When Alan visited the other day, bringing more trees, he said we had planted the first batch a bit too far apart from one another. He should know, he's been regenerating rainforests for years, but when I repeated his observation you seemed sceptical about "experts". I wanted us to fill in some of the gaps.

At first you got quietly ratty that I'd reminded you about the gaps. But I didn't insist. In no position to insist. Can't dig holes. Back won't let me. So you dig. And if you don't want to dig, digging doesn't get done. OK.

Then, quite suddenly, you changed. You agreed, ungrudgingly too, and got on with digging holes in gaps, while I planted, fertilised, mulched. Not like you at all. Stubborn, you are. I was expecting you'd continue to spread the trees too thinly. And then I would go back later and use the remaining trees to fill in the gaps as I'd originally suggested. I could probably manage to dig a decent enough hole using the pick daintily, with one knee on the ground to save my L-4 and 5 vertebrae from the brunt. So this was my plan. But it wasn't necessary to carry it out.

Judging by the way you suddenly changed tack, I think something else came into your mind other than the persuasiveness of my non-argument. Was it the realisation that you were arguing with me just for the sake of it, just to win a point? You've been doing this on and off for the last two years or so. Get the mote of what you consider our unsatisfactory relationship out of your eye, Noel. Your wanting to pursue sex and drugs and rock 'n' roll in Bangkok doesn't make Alan any less of an expert on rainforest regeneration.

I don't want you to help me with "my" projects if you don't want to. I would prefer to do things myself, in my own slow and methodical way, following the advice of people who know better than either of us. But still you help, encourage, plan ahead. Clearly part of you wants to. That's the part that shone through your resentment this morning, brightly and suddenly.

Since you were alone over my Easter retreat, you've been getting up much earlier than usual in the mornings and reading *The Tibetan Book of Living and Dying*. I looked into it today after you left for work. Your bookmark was at this quotation from the Buddha:

*Do not overlook negative actions merely because they are small; however small a spark may be, it can burn down a haystack as big as a mountain.*

## Saturday 1 May

You got up early again and went off to plant trees by yourself. I wrote. Jack away at Ben's. Out together for a meal this evening and then to see the movie *The Last of the Mohicans*. Daniel Day-Lewis, whose fine acting talent was hardly stretched in this one, looked splendid with wild flowing hair and bare chest. Fair took my breath away.

## Sunday 2 May

We finished all the tree planting today — a total of 255 trees in the ground during the last month or so. Standing back and surveying the work is very satisfying. I have a picture in my mind of how they will have jumped in about three or four years time, how they will begin to resemble a forest. We'll plant no more this year, since winter will be here soon, with the risk of frost setting them back. Also, I feel that I can manage the area we've planted — just — in terms of keeping weeds down and watering when necessary. The maintenance is definitely my job.

My physical limitations are still marked; I know them well. Between the house garden and the rainforest remnant my back will have perhaps only slightly more work than is advisable for it. Which is fine. It needs a challenge in between the resting. And I find the daily physio exercises so dull. I'm managing to maintain my current flexibility by doing the exercises about three times a week.

## Monday 3 May

I meditated for well over an hour this morning — luxury. Because you "boys" had gone off to work and school, I didn't have that sense of someone waiting for me that sometimes afflicts my early-morning sits. After that I felt a need to lie down. So I lay down. I thought about introspection and solitude, and the indulgence of this journal. I thought about the unpopular image of disappearing up one's own navel. I thought about Eliot Rosewater, in Kurt Vonnegut's *God Bless You, Mr Rosewater*, telling a convention of science-fiction writers that little bits of individual lifetimes were of no consequence compared with galaxies, eons, and trillions of souls yet to be born.

I loved Vonnegut when I was young: *The Sirens of Titan, Cat's Cradle, Slaughterhouse 5*. I wonder how I would respond to his black humour now? I've changed so much. I agreed wholeheartedly back then that the issues were eons and galaxies. I was supremely bored by the personal, and made a fetish of my ennui. Love rarely triumphed in the Vonnegut novels nor in my world. Although I felt it in my heart, I couldn't articulate it in my life, as, perhaps, I am learning to do now.

And if I am indeed disappearing up my own navel, what I am seeing there is a microcosmic universe, the thousands of facets of my own reality reflecting what Vonnegut called the "issues". As the connections that make my own reality grow clearer, so too do the issues and my ability to integrate them.

In short, unless I understand myself and my responses to life, and unless I acknowedge as much of myself as I can discover, how can I respond to others with honesty, understanding, and kindness? In this latter part of my life, this is the only response I value. In my unthinking, decidedly puzzled youth, I caused probably no more than an average amount of pain to others, especially, I think, men. I don't recall kindness ever being emphasised in ways that were meaningful. Family, school and church each had its own litany about love, goodness and charity. But living examples of these qualities were few.

I recall a missionary in Africa, a Catholic nun, advising me to "follow my heart" in making life-choices. It amazed me in its simplicity. No-one had ever suggested anything like it to me before. I know now that she was talking about fulfillment. And through fulfillment, true generosity of spirit.

People talk about the selfishness of youth as though it were something innate. Yet I wonder. It must be at least partly a consequence of living in a society where competition against others is the fundamental value. Look at the schools! Best in the class, best at this, best at that. Is any time given over to the virtues of having a good heart, regardless of one's academic prowess?

Ah youth. Jack has me wondering: how will it be for our children?

Is it possible, I wonder, ever to be a mother and feel truly free at the same time? A few days ago when I was at the Bangalow shops, one of the shopkeepers, a woman I often enjoy talking to, announced quietly that she was pregnant. She is not young. Perhaps, like me when I got pregnant for the first time, thirty-eight. Just before I left the shop she said, "I wouldn't want to have gone through life without having had the experience". I smiled.

Her words stayed with me all the way home. They bothered me. I recall thinking in much the same vein when I was trying to get pregnant, in the eleventh hour of my fertile life. And I have since heard other older women express the same sentiment. What came to me when I heard her say that, and what I could not and would not express to her just then, when she had stars in her eyes, was "The *experience*? Having a child isn't an *experience*. Your first driving lesson is an experience. A holiday on the Great Barrier Reef is an experience. But not having a child. Having a child is a change in your very perception of life. Another life will pass through your body and you will never be the same again. You will be a mother, which means by some unwritten law of the universe, that you will never again be free. An invisible cord will bind your heart to your child, and although society and good sense demand that at some point you let that child go, your heart will never let go. Even when my boy is middle-aged, I know I'll be bound by my concern for his destiny. And I'll still, out of the corner of my eye, be subtly looking for signs of the remarkable in him. And when it comes my time to die, my thoughts will turn to those moments in our lives when we both saw our own selves reflected in one another, and for a microsecond of thunderous insight we knew the infinite wellspring of love that has nourished us both through many lifetimes together. And I will die, as I think I truly shall, with my heart still bound to his."

But that's not the sort of thing I'd readily come out with in the fruit shop on a weekday afternoon.

### Tuesday 4 May

I woke at about 4.30 this morning, and got up an hour later. It's now 6 a.m. Very cool. It is still quite dark, and the mists are obscuring the river flats. So still. So beautiful. Through the study window I can see the day beginning. Jack saw a shooting star in the eastern sky last night. He got quite excited about it, saying it had a tail like a comet, which broke up into colours. I have only ever seen one like that myself. I was sorry I missed it. I had called him from his bed (he was still awake) to see a huge mist ring around the moon. He had not seen this lovely sight before, and agreed it was worth getting out of bed to see. Then as I turned to go into the house he said, "Oh, look! A shooting star!" But by then it was too late for me. "Make a secret wish!" I said. I could almost hear him making it, thinking very hard about it. "I mustn't tell you what it was, must I?" "No."

I dreamed again of a tidal wave. I've had dreams of tidal waves on and off for several years now. They are never the same dream, but all involve my seeing a wave coming, preparing for death, being engulfed, and yet somehow surviving. In this latest one I was on a steel bridge with (unknown) friends. There were huge waves, and we saw with delight masses of dolphins leaping among the waves, leaping towards us, very close. Then I saw behind them a gigantic wave that I knew would tower above us and the bridge. I took hold of the hands of the friends within reach and I intoned the words of the Buddhist *metta bhavana* practice: "May all beings be well; may all beings be happy; may all beings be free from suffering, and at peace". I remember thinking to myself that these were fitting thoughts to have in one's mind at the moment of death. I do not think I was afraid. I had no feeling of being engulfed by the water, unlike some of my other wave dreams. The next scene was my regaining consciousness in a bed in an unknown house. I was well down under the covers, where it was dry, but as I emerged and saw that everything else in the room (which miraculously had not been swept away) was wet, I realised with amazement that I had survived the wave. I wondered if anyone else had. At that point the dream seems to have ended.

As I lay in bed this morning thinking about the future of our family unit, I realised that although I now seek solitude, I fear loneliness. This came as something of a surprise. I have never really considered myself capable of feeling lonely. I have had such close loving friends in my life, probably more so now than ever, not that I see much of them, and more than half of them are overseas.

But they are not people I have shared my life with as I have with you, my husband. I have never seriously considered that your emotional attachment to me might lessen, which is what seems to be happening now. Though you tell me you will "always love me", in the sense of my happiness being of equal importance to your own, it is your *need* for me that you appear to be shaking off. Which is just what I've always said any relationship between a man and woman can well do without! Well, it seems that now is the time for my theorising to be put to the test.

## Friday 7 May

I woke up at 4 a.m. with a searing stomach pain. It was an attack (what an appropriate way of putting it) of diarrhoea. I've just had to look up diarrhoea in the dictionary. What a spelling! I would never have got it right in a million years. I don't think I've had cause to write the word before. But this last year or so I seem to have become prone to the odd bout. The last one was about three months ago. I had to cancel my creative writing class that time — unprecedented.

I've been feeling depressed all day. Can't put a finger on it, but suspect it has to do with being just plain tired of feeling unwell. It's been two years now. That vague feeling of general malaise, lack of energy, all sorts of little things going wrong physically, never feeling completely well. I've never been a wildly physically energetic person, but I've always felt well in my body. Now these little sicknesses one after the other give me the appearance of a sick person, which in my mind I know I am not at all. I don't revel in it one bit, unlike the hypochondriac who builds an identity around it.

I've just been lying down. When I got up I stared at the wall for a while, wondering what to do, not wanting to do anything. I would love to swim. It always brings me alive. But there's nowhere. Our dam is wretched with weeds and the sea is too far away and too cold by now.

I dragged myself to this desk and forced myself to write. Normally this is nowhere near so hard to do. But now at least I feel I've accomplished something, even if it is only a record of a rather miserable day.

9.30 p.m. — Now here's a thing. After writing the above I

moped around a little longer and then, since the stomach pain had subsided, decided to go into town to collect my new letterhead and business cards from the printer. I stopped off at the post office to pick up the mail. There was a lovely postcard from Julie, a Buddhist friend living in Sydney. She expressed such friendship that the day immediately looked brighter. And then there was a letter from Emma! A woman who attended our recent retreat and who at first I had found cold, distant, a pedant. I observed her gradually soften as the retreat progressed, and in the end we had some pleasant and friendly exchanges, which left me with a warm memory of her. But I did not expect such a letter; it lifted my spirits further:

> In a space of quiet reflection on a Sunday afternoon I finally get to write to you. Birds call and the tin roof creaks in the cooling rays of autumn sunlight ...
>
> I have been practising my mindfulness of breathing and newly-awakened metta meditations mightily, and find them a real source of calm and positivity ...
>
> Thank you my friend for your hospitality and energy in making the retreat possible for me and others ...

And a note from another Buddhist friend: "Although we do not see/write each other, I do think of you. Wishing you well, much love ..." Followed by a note from one of my writing students, whose work is verging on the brilliant: "I'm looking forward to seeing you again. Thanks for all your enthusiasm, skill and support ..."

These friendships with women! A new and growing thing in my life, and precious. I, who had always hung out with the boys and found women boring and uninspiring, now find I respond with warmth and pleasure to their particular ability to open their hearts.

But the cream on the cake of my resuscitated day was surely when Jack, who as you know likes to cuddle but very rarely offers verbal sentiments, said to me just before he went off to bed, and quite out of the blue, "Mum, I love you".

## Monday 10 May

The sun is coming up through a haze of mist. It's quite damp and cold, quite lovely. If it doesn't rain today I'll have to water the 255 young trees, which will take at least two hours. I must set up some kind of sprinkler system.

I'm on my own for the second day. Jack spent the weekend with his friend James. You went up to the Gold Coast yesterday morning for a friendly tennis tournament, and will stay up there for work today and tomorrow. "It'll give you the chance for a little retreat", you said, thinking I might like some time for meditation.

But yesterday I just had my usual daily sit and no more. I had planned to use the time to get some work done on the children's novel, which has been "draining" (as Kipling so aptly put it) for months. I sat at the word processor for a while reading the last chapter I had written. It inspired me not at all. I wrote about three further sentences and then left it. I put on my work gear and went off to the rainforest remnant and sprayed the weeds between the trees for about an hour. Now the rest of the mulch can be put down. I'll probably do that today.

I spent the rest of the day just lying around reading. I haven't had a day like that for a long, long time. I read newspapers and magazines mostly, some of them women's magazines that I'd got with a view to seeing if there were any to which I might contribute. But apart from *HQ*, the ones I looked at still seem to lock women into being sexual, cultural and commercial game. They might have the odd challenging and thought-provoking article, but the general package is invariably glitzy, mainstream and commercially motivated, encouraging women to be beautiful consumers.

I found it a little depressing really. But the depression wasn't entirely brought on by the women's mags. I had woken up with it. This morning was the same. There is a feeling of "Oh, another day. What am I going to do with it?". This is quite unprecedented. Though I've had low points in my life before, this feeling of hanging in a gap, of not wanting to move in any direction, is unknown to me. So I am forced to stay with the moment. My meditations should make this par for the course, but in fact they have been rather barren lately. I don't seem to have carried over the energy accumulated during the Easter retreat. Perhaps the change that you are undergoing is affecting me more than I realise.

Sometimes I feel that I am living so much between my own ears that it has become unhealthy, but it happens so naturally. Though I spent yesterday lolling around, I did give considerable thought to what I *should* be doing in order to be more "productive". Yet why should every day be "productive"? Why should I not spend some days standing and staring, even when I'm not on meditation retreats?

I'm tired of production. Production is reducing the planet to plastic wrappers and beer-can rings. We shall be smothered in it if the global population catches the work ethic.

I comfort myself in my apparent laziness with the thought, which certainly most writers would share, that creativity depends on a nice mix of laziness and hard, sometimes frenzied, work. How could it be otherwise? Even God had a rest on the seventh day.

David Malouf said in a recent interview:

*... You have to know when the right thing to do is to be patient and when to leap. You must be willing to enter into either of those situations.*

*As a writer, you must realise there will be long periods*

*when you must be patient, wait for some new idea to come, not fret about it, not push too much, say to yourself this is the time to sit patiently and wait on circumstances. It is only by being willing to drift that the other thing is going to happen.*

*You kind of say to yourself, "Basically, I cannot make a mistake, I will know the right moment, and even if I make a false move, that false move will be a necessary false move I have to make in order to make the right move later".*

*You must learn the skill of turning adversity into triumph, to come through suffering spiritually whole and somehow enhanced, or everything else will break you, and you will fail. Remember, failure comes in many guises — the simplest one is success!*

I suspect sometimes that my angst over my "laziness" comes partly from living with you, my husband. Such an obviously energetic person you are. You do lots of things, obvious things, like earning a reasonable salary and putting up fences and renovating barns. My things are not like that, yet it seems to me that I do quite a lot. I don't know where this odious habit of comparison comes from — the "I don't do as much as him, so he must think me lazy" syndrome. Maybe one day my meditations will help clarify things in that regard.

You have never really said anything to make me think that way, apart from your ongoing suggestion that I could earn more money. When we went out to dinner last Friday night you gave me a real morale boost, saying what a caring, creative mother I have been to Jack and how one can see in him the benefits of this. And you thanked me for my understanding response to your current "mid-life crisis" (your words). We talked about our friendship, our respect for one another and how we both felt it would remain firm, whether or not we stay together as a conventionally married couple. And you seemed to me to be happier than you've been for a while.

The talking about it as it happens is helping, I am sure of that. Our mutual assurances that we'll make helping one another our prime concern, rather than reacting with fear and clinging. All this—plus the dinner was excellent.

## Monday 17 May

I have been trying to get back to this journal for a week. The need to write was so strong, but the space was not available. How ironic, following those days of lazing, when I couldn't bring myself to write at all. I was teaching every day but one last week—two-, three- and four-hour classes, and enjoyed them all. My period came and went (a week early) as an almost total non-event. No PMT to alert me of its imminence; only a slight headache the day before, and tiredness. But it still surprised me. How nice. This is in great contrast to the norm of the past year or so, when my back pain has had me in its grip as an adjunct to the irritability that normally comes with PMT. The run-up to the bleeding is usually the most uncomfortable time, so I am pleased with the comparative ease of these last two or three cycles. Also this last period was very light, very little bleeding, no need to change the sheets.

I am hearing and reading more about menopause (a misnomer, since it only means the last bleed. The correct term for the entire experience, which can last anything from one to several years, is "climacteric", as Germaine Greer refers to it in her book). I've just finished *No Change* by Wendy Cooper, which is a crusade in favour of hormone replacement therapy. Its main thesis is that the reduction in oestrogen production by the deteriorating ovaries is what leads to all those ghastly menopause symptoms and that women who take HRT not only drastically reduce their symptoms, but also stay younger and sexier and consequently have happier marriages and lead fuller lives. The whole thing's written like a piece of advertising; extremely off-putting for a number of reasons. For me the greatest put-off was the slavish faith in what Cooper calls "the top men" in gynaecology.

I know a number of women who say they have benefited from HRT, and I've no reason to doubt this. What I objected to in *No Change* was the extremism and the fact that *not one other factor was mentioned*. There was nothing about individual attitude, lifestyle, diet, exercise, responses to pressures and stresses, and so on. Not even a passing nod, that I recall. Germaine Greer's *The Change* gets stuck into this particular book, saying that according to Cooper, women's happiness consists "in becoming a more exact fit to a man".

*No Change* makes no bones about encouraging menopausal women to take HRT to restore their sex drive. Where reduction in oestrogen leads to a shrinkage and drying of the vaginal tissues, obviously intercourse becomes painful. If in such a case the woman wants to continue having intercourse, I dare say it's fair enough to go for the hormone tablets. But there's no mention in *No Change* of the fact that by the time they reach middle age some women may no longer be interested in sex, some may have physically repulsive partners or sexually inept ones—any number of other factors can lead to a loss of libido. Of the women I've talked to so far, including myself, who have rather gone off sex for the moment, none has mentioned pain during intercourse. And most, like myself, love their men and do not find them repellent at all. They've just *gone off sex*. Is that not allowed in our society? In older, traditional, and arguably wiser societies, the already recognised separateness of the sexes looms even larger in middle and old age.

For me, all of this raises again the issue of how viable

the nuclear family is. Yes, yes, yes, in the context of a child needing both male and female adults (the same ones) in its upbringing, but a big NO to the idea of a man and a woman binding themselves inextricably to one another with socially, sexually, and culturally wrought chains.

I'm now half way through another book published in Britain, *Overcoming the Menopause Naturally* by Caroline Shreeve. It came out in 1986 and has been reprinted a few times. It has a remarkably different tone from *No Change*, as one might expect. She points out that in Britain fewer than two percent of patients have been willing to accept HRT because of cancer fears. Though it seems there is still a lot of controversy over this. I liked Caroline's question:

> ... *How has such confusion arisen in the first place? Either HRT involves a risk of cancer, or it does not, so how can different opinions exist over a point that is either true or false?*

While I personally don't subscribe to the "true-or-false" view of the universe, we are so often told by scientists that science is truth, and here is a scientific endeavour that has thrown up so many differing reports that even the researchers would have to doubt their methods.

Shreeve looks mostly at individual lifestyles and responses, making a case for staying involved with work and community, eating wholefoods (including a lot of raw food), getting plenty of exercise, practising a daily relaxation procedure, staying away from caffeine and nicotine, and drinking alcohol in moderation. Okay. I'm doing all that. Except the bit about raw food. I don't eat as much fresh fruit, salad or vegetables as I know I should and I probably err on the wrong side as far as processed foods are concerned. There are some I absolutely love, like crisps and chocolate biscuits.

I still need to clean up. Even though I consider I'm

doing well with my Monday fasting and cutbacks on caffeine and booze, I know in my heart that with further effort I could feel a lot better. Caroline Shreeve talks about fresh juices, with particular reference to carrot, celery and beetroot being helpful in lessening symptoms. Yesterday I determined to eat more raw and fewer processed foods, and to dig out the juicer from the box in which it's been packed since we moved from Sydney.

I had almost nil back pain yesterday and spent a day of bliss among my vegetables, weeding and tending and mulching. Jack cleaned and vacuumed inside my maelstrom of a car, doing a very thorough job for an agreed $2.50. You mowed the lawn and raked the clippings for my mulch. Thank you.

## Saturday 22 May

More insistent back pain this week. I am planning to go for a prolonged course of acupuncture for the pain relief, starting (hopefully) on Monday or Tuesday next. I also had impetigo around my left eye. I thought it was just a little itch at first, then it spread down my cheek and wept and grew angry. I took myself off to the local doctor, who diagnosed it and prescribed an antibiotic. It cleared up almost immediately. Then I wondered why I didn't go to a herbalist instead of saturation-bombing my immune system. I guess it was because I really wanted an antibiotic, knowing how quickly they work and wanting to be rid of the stigma of "skin disease" so publicly displayed.

"School sores" — I, who rarely even gets a zit! It looked repulsive. I wondered what brought it on. Perhaps Jack was the carrier, though he didn't contract it. *I* contracted it. Stress can provide it with a nesting place, as is the case with many skin ailments. Am I more upset by the current and impending changes you are putting in my path than I realise, or care to acknowledge?

## Monday 24 May

You had been away on business for a few days, returning on Saturday evening. We had a quiet dinner, the three of us. You preoccupied with your thoughts, as you have been so much lately. Hardly talking. But yesterday we talked long and hard.

You are in crisis. You are distraught. And I am experiencing a blend of compassion and bitterness. You say you want to be with us and you don't want to be with us. You admit that you regard Jack as an encumbrance, a block on your freedom, and yet you love him and feel a strong sense of duty towards him. (You took the horses out riding together in the afternoon and had a fine time. You are generally thoughtful and kind with him. So that is good.)

You say you love me, and would never wish to hurt me. But you say you are tired. You've been carrying the financial responsibility for the family too long. You want to be free to pursue other things, though you don't know what.

If I had been a serious earner, financially independent of you, would these problems have arisen? How exploited do you feel? How much does your acknowledged desire for "sex, drugs and rock 'n' roll" drive you? You're forty-two. Are you conforming to the image of the randy man in mid-life crisis? I think part of the answer is yes, and that must be where my feeling of bitterness is springing from. I feel sobered by the fear and jealousy that are arising in me.

We talked about our astrological cycles, the significance of them. I showed you what Robert Hand had to say about my current Saturn square Venus transit, and explained how powerfully I have been experiencing its lessons. I felt it was time to tell you about my passion for the physio-therapist that arose last November. "Did you have an affair?" you asked. "No." Were you hoping I'd say yes?

You said that today is the day you get the word on whether you will stay in your job or be "let go" as they so kindly put it these days. I see what a strain this has been for you and wonder how much the uncertainty has contributed to your crisis. Had I also been a breadwinner worthy of the name, your anxiety might not have reached such heights. But then again, you describe yourself as a high achiever, so perhaps work and money will always concern you.

I do not know, and neither do you. But it distresses me greatly to see you in tears, so confused, when you have been the Rock all these years. You kept saying, "It's scary, it's really scary". I can see you're not making that up. I'm scared too. More for you than me. You're not a person that's used to looking within. You've bowled through life on the currents of convention. But now convention's let you down. Your marriage contract is fraying at the edges.

I didn't suggest you learn to meditate, thinking you might find that self-serving. Instead I suggested you try hypnotherapy. You might remember I had some success with it years ago when I was having those nightmares that you used to cuddle and rock me out of. I found your reply odd. You said you didn't want your "dirty linen" displayed all over the community, mainly because of repercussions for Jack. I wonder at this. It shows such a mistrust of people, and a lack of recognition that we *all* share these kinds of problems to a greater or lesser degree. I told you it's not a question of "dirty linen"—such a bourgeois term. You seek out a professional and objective person who may be able to help clarify things for you. You said you'd think about it.

I also fear for myself and wonder at my own role in this. In my well-intentioned attempts to be compassionate

and all-giving, have I served only to increase your confusion and frustration? After telling you about my now-
defunct feelings for the physiotherapist I said, "What
about you?"

**You:** What about me?

**Me:** Yes, what about you? Any "other" women? *(my voice and
eyebrow-movement self-mocking, self-protective).*

**You:** *(Hesitant at first)* Two I'm attracted to, both divorced, both
with children. One has grown-up children. The other's young-
est is a little older than Jack. *(Pause).* I wouldn't want to be
involved with anyone with young children.

And that was it. We were quiet for a while. I didn't ask
any more. Found I didn't want to know any more. Better
not to know. Then I asked myself why, why don't I want
to know? Is it jealousy? Is that possible after all my
theorising about freedom within relationships?

In the past whenever I've asked you (never very intently)
if you were attracted to other women, you've always said
yes. Then I've said, "Anyone in particular?", and you've
invariably replied, "Everyone", and we've laughed at your
honesty. You like women, always said you prefer their
company to men's. Find men in groups rather "gross".

Then what? I asked you if these two women reciprocated
your feelings. You said you didn't know, but that some
interest had been implied in conversation, in "flirting" ways.
I fell to thinking. You going to Thailand or Bali for a few
months of freedom was perhaps something I could accommodate. But the pictures I was forming of these other
women suggested to me "relationships" rather than "just
sex". It's the kind of man you are. That's what makes it
hard for me to imagine you having an affair without getting
involved. Without, oh my God, "falling in love".

Am I romanticising you because it reflects well on me?
*My* man couldn't possibly have sex with anyone he didn't

love because he's too nice a guy. I wouldn't be involved with anyone that wasn't a nice guy, because I'm so discriminating and anyway so worthy of the love of nice guys ... and so on.

So when we discussed it again later in the evening (it was you who wanted to talk further), I found myself backpedalling from my previous *laissez faire* attitude. You said there was a possibility that if you do keep your job you will have to work one more day a week up the coast. That'll make three days and two nights a week away. You've been away from home, anyway, quite a lot lately, doing various courses, attending various meetings. I enjoy the space and I think you do too. But Jack has started complaining, mildly, about the frequent absences.

I saw your imagined relationship with the one or more women burgeoning, taking you further from Jack. I didn't like it at all. I found myself saying that if this were to happen I would be happy to remain friends, but I might find it hard to continue our sexual relationship.

At this I am both surprised and not surprised. I am not surprised because in a way I've always been one-to-one sexually; a matter of pride, I think, and a matter of not being a very sexually-oriented person anyway. A sexually-oriented woman would have flung herself at the divine physiotherapist last November, but I temper my responses. Sex has been mostly warmth and company for me. It may start as lust, but has always eventually and most importantly become warmth, comfort, belonging. So I have to admit to being unable to understand how people can risk enduring aspects of their lives in the pursuit of sex. So, bearing all this in mind, I am not surprised by my display of jealousy.

As far as my growth in wisdom and I hope, compassion, is concerned, I *am* surprised by my jealousy. As far as my criticism of the nuclear family is concerned, I *am* surprised by my jealousy. As far as my commitment to the Buddhist path of non-clinging is concerned, I *am* surprised by my jealousy.

And I'm calling to mind something one of my students wrote a while ago, describing her breakup with her boyfriend:

"'If you love someone, let them go'—cosmic bullshit!"

Well, of course you pointed out my contrariness. What else could I do but admit it? The clinging-spouse ethic is the one I was raised with. It may take more shifting than I've so far achieved by my meditations. It will take either a great deal more meditation, or it will take the actual experience of sharing my man. It could, conceivably, take both.

Seems to me that sexual relationships are in crisis everywhere. And I've long thought I knew the reasons why. Though I'm not sure that makes it any easier, for either of us.

## Tuesday 25 May

I woke at 4.15 a.m. It's now 5.45 and still dark. I like this time for writing.

I woke from a dream in which I had decided to leave you and Jack. I was to return to my parents' home and wait and see what happened. You had some serious disease, undefined. But I still felt you could cope, and that my leaving would be the best for all of us. You were surprised by my announcement, in front of friends at dinner, that I would be "leaving before 11 a.m." the following day, and if you could take me to the train station "I would appreciate it".

I thought hard about returning to my parents' poor household, of having to carry suitcases again back and forth to trains because they had no car. But I told myself

I would deal with things day by day, that it would be alright. I remembered at some point that my parents were dead, but this didn't seem to matter. I thought about being alone. The freedom. I though about going into pubs by myself, about finding my old boyfriend again. You said something about doubting if I "had the guts" to go through with it. You also gave me some information on "generating extra income", saying something like, "it's important, you know". I had vague thoughts of "showing you" — but this niggling was not the overriding feel of the dream. The theme was one of sorrow on both our parts.

The next morning I packed. You saw I was serious. You leaned back against the wall in distress. I said that it was breaking my heart to leave Jack, but that Jack loved you more than me and this was his home. I said it was a measure of my love and confidence that I was willing to leave Jack with you. I would not leave him with anyone else. I wasn't crying.

Then (I think) I woke. When I realised it was a dream the relief was immense. I thought of Jack in the room next to me and was greatly comforted. I lay in bed for a while thinking about you. No tears. I have hardly cried since the issue of living more separate lives arose. This surprises me a little.

You're away for most of this week. I appreciate it that you phone almost every day when you're away. Yesterday's call was to tell me the job decision was still dangling. No decision, not until you go to Sydney on Wednesday. With your work plus meetings for me at Jack's school, Wednesday evening was the only time we were to have together. Now that's gone. I sometimes wonder whether seeing less and less of you is a benign cosmic run-up to separation.

Another point you raised in our last talk together was that I seem to enjoy more and more being alone. "You don't need friends the way you used to", you told me. I didn't deny it. I thought about it. It is true. We have always had a lot of friends. In Sydney the house was quite busy with them. And there was Dad too. There were more people in our lives then.

I consider the strong friendships I have now, particularly with women, are far more significant to me than my friendships have been in the past. But you are right. Our lives have changed a lot as I have grown more inward. I was always the friend-getter for both of us. The few close friends I have now are my friends rather than our friends.

There's irony here. I feel I am beginning to move out of that "quieter" period of my life, as I think I've noted elsewhere in this journal, in accordance with the Saturn cycle in my astrological chart. But then, if I am to be more "active in the world", it could well be in ways that exclude you even further.

I also thought about my novel as I lay in bed this morning. If ever there was an isolating process, writing is it. I wrote a lot yesterday, even after the long entry in this journal. I am enjoying it, for the most part. Being back in the country of the imagination, following behind my characters and writing down what they say. But it is also a kind of agony. An agony of self-doubt. Will this turn out to be rubbish? I won't judge it too harshly until the first draft is finished, until I know where it has finally gone. And at the moment I have little idea where that will be. I live with the process.

My life seems to be getting fuller, and that is good. You are much in my thoughts but I cannot and do not allow our difficulties to overcome all else. Our willingness to talk to one another with honesty will be our way through. I must remember this always. I must remember that surviving with grace is what is most important to me. Not clinging. Not vendettas. Not "showing you".

Do you remember what you said yesterday morning? I'm amazed that I omitted it from yesterday's entry. Perhaps I wanted to forget it. Freudian, maybe. You told me that you had been having a "strong feeling" that you would be dead within a year or so. It made my heart drop with fear. You couldn't tell me any more, couldn't say anything further, only that it was a "strong feeling".

When I look at you, your eyes are turned inward. I have never known you like this before. You say you have never known yourself like this before. You are not here. You are no longer with us. Now I am crying.

I do not know to what extent writing all this down primes my feelings. I only know that I must write it, that I do not want the details lost.

## Thursday 27 May

You didn't lose your job. But you didn't tell me that at first when you phoned yesterday. You just told me what time you'd be arriving home. Instead of a spontaneous "Good news!" such as one might reasonably expect after all the angst over the possibility of being given the flick, all I got was a subdued ETA. I asked what news otherwise, and then you said, "I've still got a job".

Well. I didn't experience any strong feeling one way or another. I suppose I was glad for you. I suppose I am beginning to realise that it's part of your story to swim on in the mainstream of 9-to-5 for some time yet. And I wish you well. You're an ethical person. The mainstream can do with ethical people.

There was a time when I harboured thoughts of your accompanying me on another kind of journey. But it begins to look more and more as though I shall continue on my path alone, or at least not with you.

No sign from you of relief or joy in your news of still having a job. I told you this morning, "If you need to say anything to me, please say it. I don't want to be kept in the dark". You talked for a while about your ongoing confusion and then said, "I keep telling myself I'd be a fool to give up all this (our home, us) for a relationship that might not last". I said, "So there is a possible relationship, *one* possible relationship? Not just a couple of women friends, as you put it earlier?"

Yes, a relationship might develop—you care about her, do not want to hurt her or us; are in a state of total anxiety about it; think it would be easier to be a bastard and just "have a root" when you felt like it. You said I am your best friend and this was why you were telling me about it.

**Me:** Well, I guess you'll do whatever you have to do. I can't sort this out for you. Whatever you choose to do I'll try to accept as a friend, provided you maintain a loving relationship with Jack … And I don't think I want to know anything about this woman, not yet at any rate. But neither do I want to be lied to or deceived.

**You:** I haven't lied to you.

**Me:** I know. I know. I know when people are being true. I've known that since I was a kid. I know when to trust or mistrust. And I trust you.

**You:** It may never happen, nothing may come of it. I don't want to mess up any of our lives …

This leaves me with a mix of feelings. At best, a kind of elation at the possibilities of real change: of not having a lover to whom I feel I must defer; of the extraordinary freedom of being "single"; of not having to share my bed; of being able to get up at 3 a.m. and write or meditate without explaining myself; of taking holidays where I like (money permitting) while Jack stays with you in your house on the hill or else with friends, which is happening more and more now in the school vacations; of no longer cooking meat; of being "me" rather than "us"; of slapping you on the back as a friend rather than comforting you as a mother and wife—the list goes on, and I can see it continuing to grow.

At worst, I see myself lonely for you and bitter at your new happiness; frustrated when things go awry with Jack and his father is not around; socially a sore thumb because the jolly giant Noel is not with me; awkward if ever your bourgeois family comes to visit and you are living on the hill with another woman — and that list goes on too.

But look, I'll stop there. I've no wish to write more.

## Friday 28 May

Woke up this morning and looked at the back of your head. I was looking not at a man, not at an individual, but at a symbol. I was looking at a symbol of manhood. What is represented for me was protection, acquisition, support, mowing the grass and the odd cuddle. I realised that we have lost sight of the elemental in our relationship. We have lost our genius for seeing beyond what each symbolises socially and culturally. We no longer really look at one another. We pay homage to the symbols that keep the unit functioning as it is expected to function.

And the unit consists largely of things outside ourselves — the house, the land, the mortgage, the jobs, the chattels. It has deadened the fires of possibility that we once shared and forced us to unshakable conclusions about one another. It seems there is no further room for manoeuvre. The solid block that I feel in my chest this morning arises from my sentimentality. Am I sentimental? Do I tend to be swayed by feelings? Yes.

## Sunday 30 May

Yesterday was bad. I cried on waking and many times throughout the day. Through the tears I made a hutch for the ducks, and was stopped mid-job by a rainstorm. Earlier I'd told you I was feeling terrible, completely knotted inside, unable to see through the tangle of emotions. I told you I was giving myself such a hard time that I might find it difficult to be "civil" to you. I used this word because the day before you had said how amazed you were at the way some couples treat one another; "At least we're civil to one another", you said. And I had thought, "Is that all we are? Is there no more than that as far as you're concerned?" But I said nothing: I was feeling pretty much at peace.

But yesterday morning the werewolves were abroad and I thought I'd best tell you about it. As a warning to leave me alone. It was not anger. It was not blame. It was more a surfacing of that abiding sense of irony that has guided my thinking about life and my responses to it for so many years; it surfaced and wrote itself large in application to *me*, to *my* relationship. And for once I could see nothing funny in it. All I felt was fear.

When I told you this morning how awful I was feeling you hugged me close and asked if I wanted to talk. I could not respond. I felt hard and cold as iron. I did not want to make it easier for you.

**Me:** No. I don't want to talk. I don't want to see you or talk to you.
**You:** You just want to make the duck hutch?
**Me:** No. I don't want to do anything except lie down and pull the bedclothes over my head. But the duck hutch has to be made. So I'll make it.

You taped music while I worked outside, beautiful music that we have often shared. I still felt like a lump of iron. I'm not even sure if I was breathing. My back hurt and hurt. All my sorrow was accumulating there.

When the rain stopped my work I sheltered, lay on the banana chair, closed my eyes. The rain was thundering down around me, sprays of it blowing in under the patio roof. My skin seemed to harden against the cold of it, but I had a sense of warmth inside of me struggling against it. It felt like a caterpillar wanting to burst through its cocoon. I started to shake, quite literally. The sense of two opposing responses to the apparent breakdown of my marriage so strong within me. And I thought, "This is my metamorphosis". As I lay there metamorphosing I heard Jack's and his friend's loud laughter from inside the house, and I thought how unaware he was, how separate from me. But then I thought, no he's not; his laughter might not be heard at all if I were any different from what I am. What I am is in part *responsible* for the fact that he laughs as often and as loudly as he does. It was a warm thought. I needed the warmth.

But it didn't complete the metamorphosis. Still I couldn't look at you, didn't want to talk to you. My job got finished. Jack called it the "duck hunch", introducing some levity to the day.

Later you worked on far-away weeds with Jack and his friend Zach. I went out in the late afternoon. When I returned you had a fire blazing and all the dinner preparations done. We watched a video of Steinbeck's story *The Red Pony* with the boys. Then bed. I read Helen Garner. I'm not sure that I should be reading her just now.

I wonder about the compulsion I feel to write all this down. Is it my strong sense of how ephemeral life is? At times of high emotion we tend to think that it will never end, the times will never end. But they do and then we almost forget that they ever happened. Such a pity in some ways, our rampant forgetfulness. It engulfs not only the details of the events, but sometimes too the conclusions we might have come to. I do not wish to forget the details of this time. Whatever might come of it, I want to retain the facts of its coming. And perhaps years from now I'll look at this, show it to Jack, show it to friends, show it to you, and we'll feel wiser for the reading. Perhaps not even years from now. Perhaps next year. Or the year after that.

## Tuesday 1 June

Cramps yesterday and today tell me that I was probably suffering PMT on Saturday, the day of crying and shaking and suspected metamorphosis. Just hormones, eh? I don't believe it's that simple. *Nothing* is that simple.

Sunday morning we talked. We made love and talked some more. Honest expressions of love, of friendship, of not wishing to hurt. You care about this woman, that is clear. You are torn, hurting. You cried. Talked about the fear of losing us both should it "turn into an affair". For my part, I sometimes marvel at you, an honest-broker, dealing with the business of life with integrity, a steadfast man (such an old-fashioned word, steadfast, like honourable), who in this age of easily shattered marriages has chosen to lay it all before me. And I have to believe you when you say I am your best friend. If I were only your wife, you may not be talking to me in this way ...

You talked about the deception our parents' generation was guilty of. Your own parents, you feel sure now, were not happy together. But the deception went on, and along with it your conditioning. It is strong in you. Upper middle-class Protestant work and family ethic. I am freer than you. Which means, perhaps, I can ride these waves more easily. You need love, you need understanding. And I must *not* cling. If I do cling, then it is not love I feel for you. If I do cling, then my spiritual practice would be a demonstrated sham.

In the meantime, ideas come to me, ideas for teaching, ideas for writing, from all sides. I am under mental siege, typing my way through it in the elegant surmise that there exists a point of equilibrium.

## Thursday 3 June

An entirely free day in which to write. So I'm sort of circling the novel again, from a distance. It is like wanting and not wanting to call on a possible new lover, this business. Wanting so much to make that journey, but afraid the steps will falter, the journey will not be made, and you'll be left only with the ghost of your excitement. It's 9 a.m. Time to make a start.

## Monday 7 June

Rain rain rain. Flood-bringing rain. The cats are sharing a small basket, keeping one another warm in the carport. And I have what I crave: solitude.

The weekend was good; social, lively. Jack's friend Ben was here and he and Jack had their customary fine time together. Light on in Jack's room early in the mornings, quiet talk and playing with Lego. Marbles later. Lots of laughter. Then all four of us off to a fair in Mullumbimby, catching up on friends' news. Then a movie in Ballina, *Into the West*, about two Irish boys and a magical horse that carries them into greater understanding. We all loved it. You and I cried when the reformed-alcoholic father says at the end, "We're all travellers at heart, though few of us know where we're going". Jack and Ben gave it the ultimate accolade: "It was as good as *Young Einstein*!"

After the boys went to bed we talked. You told me the "other" (can't seem to attach another label) woman had given you the flick. Did not want to become lovers unless you were prepared to spend more than two days a week with her, which you say isn't an option for you.

**Me:** Are you disappointed?
**You:** Not really ... seems strange, but if anything her pronounce-
  ment has increased my resolve to spend more time away from

home. Maybe because that potential complication's been removed. I thought I'd look into cheap accommodation on the Gold Coast. Apart from anything else, my job may require me to spend three rather than the two days a week up there anyway.

Nothing new in this. We've been aware of this possibility for some time now, even before the girlfriend issue arose. So now you're talking about spending three, maybe four nights a week away. Home on Friday for the weekends. You say you may decide you don't like it. That it's crazy. Why spend time away from a loving family, congenial home? But you need to give it a try. And you need to free me up too, you said. "Sometimes I think I'm doing you a favour", is how you put it. Maybe you're right.

If you do find yourself another woman, you said you'd let me know. You said nothing will change your love and friendship for me. You said there was "no way" you would leave Jack and me in the way that so many men leave their families. All this you say and I believe you are in earnest.

All through the weekend and still today I feel calm, content with the way we are dealing with this. It's still just theorising of course. I've no real idea how I'd react to your having an affair. I don't seem to identify much with my image as a sexual being—it hardly enters into things. I identify much more with my ability to communicate my life's experience to people and with my desire to help people see things from a creative rather than reactive point of view. But whether this is strong enough to carry me through this time I do not know.

Long before my marriage I had felt that my destiny lay in areas other than making a comfortable home, living according to and advocating the marital staus quo. But I lacked the experience to really know the truth of that. Now I have the experience. But do I have any strength?

Sceptical though I am about the undue emphasis put

upon the sun signs (star signs) in pop astrology, I am aware that having the guts to go with what you know to be true is a problem for Pisceans. We lack guts. Now what can I use as a substitute for guts? Equanimity. Yes. That will have to do. At least until such time as I've grown so used to the situation that I no longer need guts to do what I must do as an individual.

To the immediate. Some pain with this period, though the bleeding is light. A lot of back pain too. Acupuncture twice a week for two weeks now. No noticeable difference. But the problem is probably compounded by the menstrual cycle. The doctor/acupuncturist also "does" Chinese herbs. He started me with them last week. I've heard good things about them from a number of women my age. So let's give it a try. Sixteen little tablets three times a day for two weeks, then we shall see. That's as well as the multi-vitamin and mineral tablet I take each day.

Hey ho.

## Tuesday 8 June

I forgot to mention in yesterday's entry that you had also said in the course of our long talk that if I, that is soon-to-be-fifty me, found myself with another lover, you would appreciate my being honest about it. Agreed. You also said, "No lovers in the house, though. Not with Jack around". Agreed. I wouldn't have thought that last point even needed discussion. But I appreciate and share that particular concern.

## Tuesday 15 June

Today I looked for a word that best describes my present state of mind. The word that occurred to me was unhappy. I do not think I've ever applied that word to myself before—not definitively. I feel unhappy. I feel bereft. Yet in that there are happinesses. Today an elderly (in her seventies) and talented student of mine said she feels as though my teaching had "blown a wind of fresh air" through her mind. And yesterday Jack and I started to make the papier-mâché landscape for his Lego castle. "This is going to be a filthy landscape", he said (meaning "great", as I understand it, in current kids' jargon).

Feeling bereft and unhappy over you. Yet if anything you're more solicitous of my needs than ever. Solicitous and at the same time pleased and excited at the prospect of your greater freedom. I sense that you are full of anticipation. So, in a way, am I; perhaps even more so.

My daily meditation practice, such as it is just now, is doing little for me in terms of insight into my current situation. The best I am getting from it is a degree of calm, of relaxation. And that, of course, is welcome.

I have talked to no-one about us, except, obliquely, to Margaret when we had lunch a few weeks ago. If Chittaprabha were here, I would share it with her. As it is, I'm not very inclined to phone. That's alright, anyway. It's you and I who are talking about it. That's all I need right now.

You said you wanted to talk to Louise, the work-friend whose place you stay at when you're up the coast. You want to ask Louise if it's OK to stay an extra night, to tell her that you and I have agreed to give one another more freedom, more space, and this may involve either of us having another sexual partner. You told me that if you do end up in another sexual relationship you don't want Louise and other people at work saying you're a bastard, that you're cheating on your wife. Well, fair enough. Ironic that these work friends of yours so recently dubbed us "the ideal couple".

**You:** I want to be straight about whatever may happen. I don't want to play games. I'm not very good at playing games anyway.

You always did have an original turn of mind. Perhaps none of this is very startling in this sexually-liberated age. I don't know. But I do admire your honesty. And I think I also understand this need you feel for more freedom. I have after all felt it myself from time to time throughout our marriage. I certainly did last November.

## Sunday 20 June

I am beginning to feel the lightness of a new freedom. I am growing in confidence in myself and my own view of things. I am noticing small changes in the way I speak to you. None of this is deliberate, or particularly startling. But I know that in the last few weeks I have been more forthright in communicating my thoughts, feelings, opinions. There is a greater clarity in the way I am expressing myself, as though I wish to leave no room for misunderstanding.

I see that you are still very much immersed in your own thoughts, and I am not asking you to share them. If you want to, we'll talk. You've told Louise that you'll be staying for at least another night up the coast, and you've told her why. She was concerned that I might feel she was the "other woman" — or rather potential other woman, since this is still basically an hypothesis in your mind. I phoned her and put her mind at rest, telling her I knew she was not because you had told me, and I know you don't lie. I told her my main concern was Jack — rumours flying that his parents had separated, which, anyway, is not the case. Told her you wanted greater freedom, most notably freedom to have another sexual relationship. Told her it was supposed to be reciprocal. Told her we want to maintain our friendship and love, our home and family. People may not understand this. So we would like if possible to keep it contained. Louise said she understood, though was surprised. She is a kind person. I think I trust her.

In the meantime, I have booked into a meditation retreat

for the first week of the next school holidays. It will not be with the Friends of the Western Buddhist Order and it will be my first retreat without Chittaprabha. Jack will be off with friend Ben and family, who have won a holiday for six at Hamilton Island for a week. You will be working up the coast for the usual two days, then away for a seminar. I've booked the dog into the kennels and Keri will do the chooks and cats. Looking forward to the break and the lack of distraction from serious sitting. And for the October school holidays I'm planning to go to Sydney with Jack. He's been invited to stay with the Elliot family and I'll stay with Chittaprabha. Almost two whole weeks together! And, joy, there will be a short meditation retreat in the middle, which Chittaprabha and I plan to attend.

Since you haven't been interested in going away together as a family—we have had only one short camping trip in two-and-a-half years—I have now stopped suggesting it. I've decided to accept your disinclination. Perhaps you're right. I am not sure that we would enjoy each other's company enough, or have enough to say to one another, to make a holiday together quite what it should be.

As this "wind of fresh air" blows through our marriage (to use Ann's metaphor), I see that it may be better for all of us if you and I spend more of these blocks of time apart, doing what interests us. Then at those times when we are together, we shall be refreshed. And I say to myself, "Let him have the time, the space, the freedom. Let him have all of next week and two weeks in October when he won't feel obliged to come home. Time to spend in the company he feels he needs right now. And if he decides he wants even more of that company, so be it. If he doesn't want it after all, so be it". I can accommodate the changes.

Meantime I see you, thinking, thinking, thinking. Not happy. And I wonder—will I leave you behind?

## Wednesday 23 June

Another long talk last night, instigated by me asking you how you were doing, how you were *really* doing. We found ourselves running about parallel, which was good. Both still feeling in a state of suspension, but generally calmer, as though growing accustomed. I ask myself this morning — accustomed to what? And I think the answer must be to our own honesty with one another.

We talked a bit about when we first met, our lives together, what we have gained from one another, what we feel we might have lost by being together so long. As far as the loss is concerned, it seems very little. I said I thought we were both fortunate in having high self-esteem — surely half the battle when negotiating stormy times in a relationship.

We talked about sex. I said I thought it was inevitable that a monogamous couple should cease to spark after so many years. Why should that be such a big deal? Seems quite normal to me. You didn't say anything. Perhaps you don't agree? Perhaps none of this would have come about if I had remained the lover that you wanted.

You remarked that the acid test of all our good faith would be when one of us comes home and tells the other we've had sex with someone else. I asked if that was still a possibility with your friend who had given you the flick (to use your expression). You said you thought it was, and that you had arranged to visit her last Monday evening, but when the time came you hadn't felt well and had gone off to bed early at Louise's place.

**Me:** You arranged the visit with sex in mind?
**You:** No. Just to talk. But I guess that might have happened. Or it might not. I may have to see what other talent is available.

Bit of a bold statement, that last one. Pushing the barriers?

I told you that if and when you do come home with the news of a new lover I would probably be happy for you. I meant it. It was heartfelt. To what extent I can boast this largesse just because you are not threatening to leave/ abandon/cut-off-without-a-penny Jack and me, I don't know. But clearly the economic factor has much to do with the acrimony that characterises a lot of marriage breakups. But I feel relatively secure, in material terms; confident that you would not leave us, or demand to sell our property and take your half. It could be my sense of security is resting on a delusion. If so, I'll need to deal with that too when the time comes. One step at a time.

Though I told you I'd be happy for you if you found a lover, I also told you — I think for the second time — that if it were to happen I probably wouldn't want to have sex with you. "I don't want to risk a disease", I said. (I'm editing a book about AIDS at the moment.)

I asked you if you would *want* sex with me if you found yourself another lover. You thought you would. I really don't think I would mind if you didn't, provided you still loved me as a friend and that the warmth and hugs continued. Maybe I'll look back on these entries in a few months (weeks? days?) and think "what rot!".

You asked (again) if there were any men I was interested in.

**Me:** No. Though I don't entirely rule out the possibility.
**You:** It would be ironic if you were the first one to come home with the news—not that it's a race (*you added hastily*).
**Me:** I didn't imagine it was.
**You:** What would bother me, would be why. (*I took this to mean that you wouldn't understand why I would take another lover when I had lost interest in sex with you.*)

I could only answer by saying that currently and for the last year or so I've had very little interest in sex with you.

But my feelings for the physio last year taught me that I can still surprise myself when it comes to romance. So how can I rule out the possibility of that happening again?

With all this re-structuring (your word) going on in our relationship I had to tell you that some of my gears were inevitably being shifted. In theory we are both acquiring more freedom. That makes me look at the world a little differently — and perhaps at men a little differently, too.

**You:** Would it be spite, getting back at me?
**Me:** I can't imagine myself having sex with someone out of spite — credit me with the self-esteem and the goodness of heart, please. But my being attracted to and attracting someone else is perhaps more likely to happen now than it was previously, now that change is in the wind.

All this, and pre-menstrual too. Due to start around the weekend, judging by the signs. Are the Chinese herbs keeping me from hurling your mother's crystal at you?

Still watching my diet. Hardly any caffeine. Hardly any alcohol. Lots of fruit and vegetable juice, and more raw food. The daily multi-vitamin and mineral tablet. And — bliss — I've started swimming. Getting to the heated indoor pool in Ballina around two or three times a week, in the early morning when it's empty. Less discomfort in the back due partly to the exercise, I'm sure.

## Wednesday 14 July

Three weeks since I've written in this journal. It seems the experience of deep peace disinclines me to write. I spent the whole of the meditation retreat on the mindfulness of breathing. No other practice. This was it. The entire retreat. Breathing. And a little yoga. No puja. No incense, candles, flowers. No eye-contact or snatched smiles over breakfast.

Just me and my breath. Eleven hours sitting a day. Stark. Zen. Just over the Queensland border.

At first I thought I'd go home. For the first two days I looked for what wasn't there, for what I was used to. Then I started to notice what *was* there and I finally grew accustomed to the differences in approach, to the starkness. And I felt glad to be among Zen practitioners.

I came away, as usual from a retreat, feeling that perhaps not much had happened after all, that I was the same old me. On the way home, the friend I was giving a lift to said, "Your driving's much slower now than when we drove up". We laughed. She was right. It is often other people who notice most.

You made it clear to me several days later that you'd been watching me quite closely. "Since you've come back from the retreat you've been so calm, so strong", you told me. "Much more so than usual. Even when we got the bad news about the house in Sydney (which we still own, and have let), you just moved through all that as though it shouldn't affect you personally. You seem so complete. It's marvellous. And coming home after the peace of the retreat and having Oliver and then his family here, and then going off to a twenty-first birthday party that you didn't really want to go to, yet being so serene about it. It's great."

Now you are not a person given to such effusive pronouncements. I smiled to myself. A Zen smile. Zen lessons. Life is *now*. Life is nowhere else but *now*. We cannot undo what has been done and we cannot tell what might be, and we are wasting our resources, to say nothing of making ourselves unhappy, if we let ourselves become obsessed with past or future.

And then ...

A few days after that, you asked me to teach you the basics of my meditation practice. We sat by the fire and I talked you through the various stages of the mindfulness of breathing. Remember you can meditate anywhere — on a train, a bus, at the beach. Don't get too precious about where and how you sit; don't get too caught up in technique. The technique is the vehicle, not the actuality. The actuality is sitting; sitting with yourself, observing yourself. This is how you bring your whole self into being. The actuality is *now*.

In the time since your first lesson you've purposefully sat quietly a few times — in armchairs, at your desk, and the other day I interrupted you lying back in the bath doing the mindfulness of breathing.

You are away now, up the coast. The new regime of overnighting two nights a week has started. Jack said last night, "I don't really miss him being away on Tuesdays as well". Jack's life is quite full. He doesn't seem to miss you in the way that that word usually implies. We talked a bit about it. I told him I liked the time away from Dad, I thought it was good for both you and me to have some separateness in our relationship. I have interests and pursuits that Dad doesn't share and vice versa. I said I was glad you had some friends of your own up the coast. Said you had let me be the friend-getter for both of us for many years.

We did some more work on the papier-mâché landscape for his Lego castle yesterday. And he asked questions about God:

**Jack:** If God is supposed to have made everything, who made God?
**Me:** I don't know, Jack. I asked the same question when I was a kid, but nobody had any answers, not even the church people. They just said it wasn't for us to ask such questions in the first place. But they never knew how to stop children asking them; they still don't. They continue to make statements, like saying that God made everything. But that automatically makes you ask more questions. Then they tell you to be quiet. It's fascinating to let your imagination go back to possible beginnings of time, the birth of galaxies and solar systems. But I prefer not to speculate about who

or what made everything. We can't even say if everything was "made" in our sense of the word. I don't think we can talk about such things for certain. Our perceptions are very limited. A frog sees a different world to us, and a dog smells a different world to us. Who knows how much of reality we are missing? All we can know about, and have some control over, is the moment now.

**Jack:** And they say God is all-powerful. So why does He let people kill one another and hurt one another?

**Me:** That's another question I asked as a child. Probably every child asks it. Some people say God gave mankind free-will, but how can there be an all-powerful God alongside creatures with free will? There are contradictions all around us, Jack. Adults make out to kids that they've got it all worked out. But most of them know doodly-squat. The universe is filled with questions, with strangeness. The Christian scriptures are filled with them. But the churchmen's way of dealing with questions is to ignore them by saying THIS is definitely so and THIS is definitely not so, THIS is definitely right and THIS is definitely wrong. It's politically comfortable, but it ties people in knots. No all-powerful God will take care of your sense of what's right and wrong. When you look at your own reasons for doing the things you do, *really* look at your own motives, you'll know.

I have started doing a little yoga each day alongside my physio exercises. I have been doing my first shoulder stands in two years, since my back injury.

### Sunday 18 July

Alone again. You left yesterday for last night's big office party, and to stay on up the coast till Wednesday. Jack is away with horse-riding friends, pony and all. My solitude is delicious. If I didn't feel obliged to put in a few hours at the working bee at Jack's school this afternoon, the deliciousness would be complete. Yesterday morning I swam, early; then tackled weeds in the rainforest remnant;

thought a bit about the renovations to the barn, about the community purpose it might serve.

Ron has taken a look at the site in the middle of the rainforest remnant where I plan to put a meditation sala — eventually.

My period is due any minute. I have had very little PMT. I do believe the Chinese herbs are helping. The doctor has said he will also give me herbs to regulate the cycle — I have been creeping back to a 21-day cycle over the last few months, in spite of the chaste berry I've been taking. The bleeding has been light, but given the PMT and the increased back pain that accompanies it, I'd rather it happened less frequently than every three weeks.

My experiment in teetotalism lasted a month. A record. I'm now back on the odd drink. Even so, after just a couple of ports the other night I had a slight headache the following day. I generally get a bit of this when I'm pre-menstrual, so that's probably what it was. But, but, but, I didn't have a pre-menstrual headache last time I was pre-menstrual, when in the grip of teetotalism. In fact I had no PMT at all. The bleeding took me by surprise. Ah ha!

You have been more relaxed of late. Your face has smoothed out a bit. You are less preoccupied with what's going to happen to us all. You say this is due to me. You saw how I was on returning from days of intensive meditation and decided that living in "the now" is kinder to the self. Which of course it is.

You're no longer just talking about the suffering that comes with change, you're talking about the excitement. You've lost weight, deliberately, and are looking the better for it. Reminds me of the state I was in last November/ December, taking extra care with the way I looked because of my fantasy liaison.

We talk so much more easily now. It is as though shedding the sexual commitment has opened up long-lost pathways of communication:

"Sure, you do that if that's what you want to do" rings through the living room ...

"I'll probably do this though ... you don't want to come? That's fine ..."

"Take all the freedom you want so long as you're here for Jack and me when we ask you—*especially* when we ask you ..."

"I am. I will be. I love you ..."

You spent all last Saturday jack-hammering inconvenient blocks of concrete out of the barn floor in preparation for the plumbing and flooring of what is part of my meditation retreat vision. Jack-hammering wastes a body. This I know, it being one of the two things I did (exactly two years ago) that drove my vertebrae into one another. I could never go jack-hammering again. So I thanked you. Particularly, I added, since my retreat vision is not a shared vision. "Let's see what happens ..." you said, meaning what? Is there a chance it *may*, one day, be a shared vision?

Do I need you? Yes I do. Although you've said I don't need anyone. You earth me. I need earthing. I need your friendship. But I don't want to be "married" to you any more. Marriage has meant trying to make one another what each felt a spouse should be. Not to the extent we see some couples doing it, but still it has happened with us. Being lovers has in some ways blinded us to what else each has to offer. Instead of accepting ourselves as we are, the possessiveness of sexual love makes us want to take more from one another. Also, paradoxically, to give more. To mould into shape. To make comfortable and predictable.

You're younger than me. You're still viewing yourself as a sexual being. Then be one. If I cannot accommodate that idea, we lose whatever else there is between us—and that is a lot. I told you that we were re-writing our Book of Marriage. We'll find something else. Don't know what we'll call it. Not marriage. Love, perhaps.

## Saturday 24 July

Today is day twenty-nine of my menstrual cycle. The bleeding still hasn't started, though it's felt imminent all week. It's a while since I've had a "normal" length cycle. Perhaps this is the effect of the Chinese herbs?

All week I've been experiencing PMT. I've heard women say this is our most psychic time in the cycle, but I don't feel that at all. Although my dreams are more vivid than usual at this time, in terms of daily living I feel as though I've shut down, I've ceased any kind of communication with my environment and my companions. I'm a completely enclosed system, intent upon itself and its own shortcomings and its own pain.

For the first time since the retreat, the back pain became an issue again this week, to the point of putting me off doing my exercises and yoga. I think the pressure build-up at this time in the menstrual cycle is what exacerbates the back injury — indeed exacerbates anything that might be dysfunctional! As far as I expect anything, I expect that when I finally stop menstruating, the back problem will in turn become less noticeable.

I had a visit this week from a friend who is experiencing early menopause. She is only forty, has been suffering hot flushes, mood swings and very heavy bleeding for two years. She knows I've been talking to a lot of menopausal women and have done a lot of reading. She wanted to talk. Once again it struck me what an individual thing the menopause is. Everyone I've talked to or read about has a different story to tell, though there are a few common characteristics — most notably feeling different within oneself, sensing that this is a major turning point; also the lack of energy, and sadly the loss of confidence (which for my money is due more to society's ignorance of and negative response to menopause than to the condition itself).

So we talked. While my symptoms are mild compared

with hers, I was able to share with her a few stories from other women I know. She was particularly interested in alternative remedies that have helped others, and to hear that evening primrose oil is available in bulk and cheaply from a local naturopath. I told her about the Chinese herbs, how I was regulating my diet to include more raw food and at least one glass of fresh-squeezed carrot/celery/beetroot/apple/orange juice a day in any combination, but always including the celery for the joint pains I have (also associated with menopause). Cutting down on alcohol and caffeine — still going OK there, all things considered. Drinking plenty of water (from our rain tank). And exercise. Still happening regularly when I don't have the pre-menstrual backache; but even then I still swim. Driving into town at least twice a week in the early mornings and doing laps for about half-an-hour.

This morning I swam and on returning home did my exercises and some yoga straightaway. Being pre-menstrual I was not as flexible as I've been these last few weeks; I just took it to that point of effort that is not punishing, and as a result felt better than I'd felt in days. Clearly some degree of pushing oneself is necessary at these times; and the benefits are felt immediately.

My forty-year-old friend also pointed this out. When she's feeling really low, she said, the last thing she wants to do is to be physical. But in fact she finds that if she forces herself to get out and do some bike-riding (which she loves), she invariably comes home feeling invigorated both physically and mentally. Much better able to cope, in other words. It's almost a truism, isn't it? Yet it seems to be something we've lost sight of, sitting in our little offices or units letting our bodies lose that sense of completeness that is our natural state.

There are *reasons* why menopause happens the way it does. Yet we're not encouraged to listen to or connect with them. We're encouraged to keep them under wraps; ignore them; suppress them; whatever. Is it the sexual connection that gives rise to this insidiousness? Is it possible, for example, that the loss of libido happens because women of fifty (the ball-park age) are no longer equipped physically and no longer inclined emotionally to have babies? And that in those few years when ovulation is slowing down the reduction in sex drive is our natural contraceptive?

Does the energy and the sex drive return afterwards, my friend asked me. Yes, according to Germaine Greer and various women I've talked to, one of whom (like Margaret Mead) defines her present blooming as "post-menopausal zest".

## Sunday 25 July

You're sitting in the living room reading *Seeking the Heart of Wisdom* by Joseph Goldstein and Jack Kornfield. I gave it to you after our conversation at the Spanish restaurant. Because it's one of the best, clearest and most inspiring books on meditation I've come across. This is what we said last night, while eating tapas:

**You:** It's not so easy, staying in the present moment, is it?
**Me:** No. Nobody said it was. The Buddha didn't promise a rose garden.
**You:** The woman I told you about ...
**Me:** The one that gave you the flick?
**You:** Yes. She told me this week she wanted to spend more time with me. But she's unhappy about the arrangement I've made with you to spend most of my time at home.
**Me:** What made her change her mind about being lovers?
**You:** I don't know.
**Me:** So you've got to this point in your discussions with her and you still tell me this relationship is not physical—not even a little kiss?
**You:** Not even that. It's not my doing that it's not physical. It's

hers. She's very conventional, very cautious. She's holding back on the physical until I make more of a commitment.

**Me:** What was your response?

**You:** I told her, sorry, I'm not prepared to do that.

And me? How did I respond to your news? Well, I accepted your confidence with neither pleasure nor displeasure. I was grateful for your trust, your honesty.

We touched one another a lot last night. Hands across the table. Arms around the neck. Some laughter. How can we live together for so many years without taking parts of one another's hearts? Even couples that hate one another are bound in some kind of heart connection — and always will be. That binding is what makes acrimonious divorce so painful, even years after. They have rejected parts of themselves.

**You:** You're very strong, you know. In a quiet sort of way. And your strength is growing.

**Me:** Was it hard saying you wouldn't spend more time with your new friend?

**You:** Not really. Which makes me think that maybe there wasn't much there anyway—in the friendship. She would have to be some woman to make me want to spend more time with her than with you.

**Me:** Thanks.

**You:** What about you?

**Me:** Me?

**You:** You and men? Are you interested in anyone in particular?

**Me:** At the moment—no. Maybe it's the menopause. Maybe it's just me. Maybe it's my meditation practice. It's probably all of those. But the way I view myself has changed. So has the way I'd like people to see me. And people includes men. I was always happy that men found me sexually attractive. But now, it's not even an issue. Think me nice looking, by all means—statuesque was how Ken put it recently and I liked that; I liked the distance it suggested. Yes, admire me because I'm statuesque. But leave my knickers alone. The most important thing now, and I would have liked some role-model to have suggested this to me when I was in my cringing pubescence, is that I be honest. Now it's possible—just possible—that I've not been entirely honest in my sexual relations, that I've run with the crowd in this regard. I don't know yet. I'm still looking at that one.

It was an interesting dinner.

Today I've been thinking about how our society makes sex a commodity; something to be bought and sold, stamped with legalities; something which attaches to profit and loss on the part of the user. How to be honest when you're always weighing up what you might get out of a situation? Witness my silly behaviour around the physiotherapist last year. Why couldn't I just tell him I liked him instead of giving him come-ons, taking my meditation stool to show him on a pretext about my back. I knew he'd bite the bait and we'd get all meaningful together about meditation ... and so on and so on.

Please, please, please ... never again.

## Monday 26 July

This was a day of weakening resolve. Also of amusement at the weakness. My period still hasn't started. I want it to start. I want to get it over with. I am a boiler about to burst. I am a bundle of extraordinary possibilities. But I am quite without direction. And in pain. I think I can say just now that none of this seems to matter much. I'm cool. I'm alright. At least I'm not causing anyone else any suffering.

It is day thirty-one of my cycle. Something different is happening. Thus far, in all my years of fertility I have only missed one period (apart from during pregnancy), and that was sometime last year or early this year. Is this a missing one? Or just late?

## Tuesday 3 August

It's day thirty-nine of my cycle and my period still hasn't happened. I went to a gathering on menopause last week. There were a lot of women there, including a few friends. Various people talked about their experiences; practitioners talked about their treatments, alternative and mainstream. It was highly informative, and for me served mainly to underline how very individual the responses to ageing can be. It was heartening to realise how much more information and networking is available than when my mother was experiencing menopause, and how openly women are talking about it. Well, middle-class women anyway.

Hey ho. And my back? Much better than it was while I was "pre-menstrual", even though there was no bleeding. That phantom period has passed and left my back in relative peace. I did a lot of physical work on the land over the weekend and it felt great.

You and Jack went riding on Sunday and Jack came back flushed with success: "I've finally mastered cantering, Mum!" Great excitement. But he mentioned later that he had an ache in his "grind". We told him "groin". But he seemed disappointed, preferring his own word.

The drainage pipes and the cement floor are down in the barn and the plumber will come again to hook up the water. Then, after I've done some cleaning and patching up, Ron will work on finishing the interior walls. It's good to have Ron's advice and his time. He is so friendly, so focussed, and he doesn't charge a packet: "If it's for the Buddhists, I'll do it!"

You are still reading *Seeking the Heart of Wisdom*. Yesterday I saw you pack it in the suitcase you take up the coast. You've just phoned from there. Said you'd had a sit at the beach.

You've been sitting in meditation most mornings for about twenty minutes. You're still asking a lot of questions about meditation and Buddhism. Jack said recently, "Maybe Dad will become a Buddhist!". How directly children voice those fragile thoughts we dare not fully acknowledge!

The other day, after you'd got back from your two nights up the coast, I asked, "Did you see your girlfriend?" You smiled. "Yes. We talked a bit."

"Was it friendly?" You smiled some more. "Yes. It was quite pleasant."

"What are you smiling at?" I asked.

"At you", you said, "calling her my girlfriend". I laughed too, and you gave me a cuddle. It was a nice exchange.

## Sunday 8 August

You sat in meditation twice yesterday—once for about twenty minutes after getting up in the morning; and then again for about half an hour before we went out to a local restaurant for dinner.

I had a visit from a fellow Buddhist from the Sydney community. I had not met her before. We liked one another immediately. She came to lunch on Friday and then went to my little cabin for a sit. She came back yesterday and meditated for the whole afternoon, following which you plied her with questions about meditation. I enjoyed listening to her answers, which were very considered. Sufficient to get you to see what an evolving phenomenon meditation is, that one cannot say "meditation is this" or "meditation is that" and consider one has dealt with it. The meditative state has very little to do with technique, or with aiming at a certain point, it is about you, the meditator; and all this becomes clearer and clearer over time. Another point that our friend from Sydney made was: "There's nothing like being unhappy to make you want to change".

You commented on this before we got out of bed this morning, and you added: "I feel as though I've undergone more personal growth in this last month or so than I have in years. The irony is that while your Buddhism and meditation was originally part of the wedge that came between us, it's now becoming the instrument that brings us closer than we've ever been."

I see how you are happier to be with Jack and me. The grumpiness has largely disappeared. You talk to me openly about the women at work that "try to race you off", about your "girlfriend".

You said that while you were up the coast last week you talked with her about "the situation". You saw it was making her very unhappy that you could not agree to giving her more of your time, so you said it may be a good idea just to cool it for a while. I'm not sure what you meant by "cool it" and I guess I forgot to ask.

When we were talking about how our friendship has grown as a result of all this, you said that you felt our growing closer doesn't make it less likely that you will form another relationship, in fact it makes it more likely. Well, there you are. I've always been fond of irony. Life is full of it. If we can accommodate it we have a far greater chance of reaching that point of equanimity from which a creative and constructive approach to life may spring.

You said you didn't know, of course, whether *the* relationship will be with this "girlfriend" — clearly there are already difficulties there. But you joked about the irony of me, your wife, giving you "the strength to have other relationships".

I appreciated the confidence, but felt I had to point out that all this was still largely theoretical — assuming you're not lying about the sex, which is what I do assume. As a result of your growing meditation practice, you seem thoroughly engaged with the present. (And you've just poked your head around the study door, asked if I want a cup of Ecco, and told me you've just had your sit and how right our friend from Sydney was about the morning being the best time.) Perhaps your girlfriend finds this odd and rather frustrating. You want to have the relationship and not think about the future structure; she, clearly, is looking ahead. I can understand her point of view.

I wonder if by placing yourself so steadfastly in the present you are not over-reacting to the lessons of meditation — taking in too much too soon. Seasoned meditators talk of the "honeymoon" period. For many people, including me, the initial encounter with meditation sends a hurricane through the mind. You have in your head the possibility of change, of clarity, direction, fulfillment, happiness — and it can happen that your embrace of it becomes too grasping. Then you start to lose it, and the realisation sets in that you require years of work to dismantle your conditioning. And you see the path is not completely strewn with rose petals after all. If you can't fill these troughs, these gaps, with faith in what you have already learned, in the changes you have already accomplished, you will abandon the path.

## Tuesday 10 August

Some moments: at coffee yesterday, Christie, the clever writing student who will surely be published one day, said, "You're important to me, an older women that I admire so much". Walking back to the house from the wilderness paddock last Sunday, Jack put his cool-dude-ten-year-old arm around my waist. We walked all the way home with our arms round one another, not saying a word. Later that day, when he and you were outside, I heard him say, "Dad, do you think I'll grow up to be like you? ... I hope so". Then Margaret phoned, in a rush, and said: "I just wanted to say hello and I love you".

## Thursday 12 August

I feel I have to make this line of words, and see where it goes. See if the words that end each sentence will illumine the ones that begin the next. That's the way of writing, of almost forcing yourself to get something on the page.

You finally "came home with the news" last night, broke it so quietly, so circumspectly. We were sitting up talking after Jack had turned in. You said you wanted to have a look at your astrological transits again. You'd been summoned to a "big" meeting next week with the powers at work. I had been looking at both our transits yesterday morning (not, I am sure, coincidentally) and was able to tell you that work should be a bit more relaxed.

I saw that there was more than work on your mind. I had seen yesterday that transitting Jupiter was only one degree off squaring your natal Venus. There is great potential for freedom, pleasure, new romantic relationships in that. On Monday afternoon you had phoned me from work and we'd had a long conversation about the stages of our respective minds. In some ways, it was the furthest we had gone in expressing our trust, our faith, our lack of jealousy. And it is what prompted me to look again at the astrological correlations. For you at the moment the only really significant transit is the Jupiter square Venus. In *Planets in Transit* Robert Hand says that this can be a time of needing to express love to others, a time when there is a strong possibility of attracting a person with whom you could have an important, if somewhat rocky, relationship. He says that although you may not appreciate it at the time, the difficulties inherent in this relationship will lead you into greater "wisdom and maturity".

Jupiter-Venus contacts often signify a clash between a love of freedom and a need for closeness with others. This particular transit can also lead to a certain compulsiveness, with the possibility of overwhelming your new partner. Proceed with caution, Hand advises, and there is a good chance you will form a relationship that is constructive for both.

So here was a cosmic possibility that was now at my

doorstep. Consequently, last night when you said to me, quietly and with no sign of discomfort or awkwardness, "Thank you again for your understanding ...", my heart did a lurch because I knew what was next, "... It finally happened last night ..."

I said, "What made her change her mind?"

You said, "It wasn't her. It wasn't 'the girlfriend'."

Relief. I felt relief. Why? Do I not want you involved? Do I grant you only casual sex?

You said it was a woman you've known for a while but had "not particularly lusted after". She had been away on holiday and when you saw her on Tuesday you suggested seeing a movie together that evening. Then you went back to her place. You didn't stay the whole night. You had an early appointment on Wednesday and your things were all at Louise's house.

**Me:** What time did you get to Louise's?

**You:** About 1.30 a.m.

**Me:** Was Louise curious? (*Why did I want to know these details? I reminded myself of a fishwife.*)

**You:** Everyone was asleep. And Louise's never curious.

I listened. Calm. Nodding my head every now and then. I had a few more questions. Just a few. You didn't mind. We were civilised. We were friends. "Was it good?" I asked. God. Why did I ask that? You said yes, though a little awkward, not being "used to" one another. I understood that. After so many years of monogamy.

**Me:** Would you go back?

**You:** Would I go back—yes. Will I go back—I don't know.

A subtle distinction. You are growing in subtlety. I've noticed this. You said she is recently divorced, kids grown. She has few constraints, unlike you.

Condoms? You hadn't used them. It wasn't premeditated, you said. And she had assured you it wasn't necessary. You then said to me that you would use condoms if I wanted sex with you—for my protection.

My immediate thought was no, why should *I* be the one that puts up with condoms? Then I thought let's stick to what I said before: while you've got a lover I don't want to have sex with you, at least not at first. Maybe later, when I'm more used to it and after you've had the necessary test(s), we'll be lovers again. But not just yet. And that's what I replied. It was actually a stronger thought than the first one. And I was glad of that.

You nodded your acceptance. We grinned. We talked about "not feeling married any more". "Bizarre", you said. "Mmm ..." I said.

We cuddled up in bed that night, as we always do. These winter nights are cool. You are always warm.

### Friday 13 August

At the swimming pool this morning when the two "old ladies" (as I think of them, even though they're probably no more than sixty) arrived, I asked them the time, since I needed to get back home earlier than usual. One of them pointed to the clock and said, "I think that's right, isn't it?" I told her I didn't know, because I couldn't see it, I didn't have my lenses in. "Oh you poor kid", she said kindly. And me nearly fifty.

My period started this evening. Thought it might. The back pain's been an issue for a few days; fortunately very little PMT, only a nagging sense of what Tim Winton in his storm-tossed *Cloudstreet* calls the Shifty Shadow of God. I kept dropping spoons, breaking needles and bruising hips, none of which carelessness is as nasty as losing four fingers (as Sam Pickles did in *Cloudstreet*).

## Monday 16 August

A weekend of activity—half crippled in the back by the time yesterday evening came round, but happy. Swirling around at a bush dance on Saturday night with you, Jack, Keri, Ted, and a number of other friends. The first time I've danced in over two years. The back allowed me. The band was a treat—bearded ferals and other earth-lovers. Virginia reels, stripping the willow, curtseying and all the rest, even a Russian dance where we all yelled "Hai!"

Yesterday was spent around the rainforest remnant: weeding, planting, nurturing, burning rubbish. I begin to see some beauty peeping through. All sorts of natural regeneration taking place after two years of not having cattle wandering through it.

We meditated together this morning. Remember?

## Saturday 21 August

A new identity is forming around me. Or is it inside me? I am watching it almost objectively. It has very little to do with my sexuality. Though that delicious feeling has not entirely gone from my life. I felt a warm sweetness pass through me yesterday as I sat beside Matthew, a big man, quiet, thoughtful, with gentleness in his eyes. I like him. I like him in a different way from the way I like my women friends and acquaintances, because he is a man, and a beautiful one at that.

Easier to tell them they're beautiful when you're nearly fifty, and you know that they know it's not a come-on. Fifty. What an honourable ring it has about it. You can't mess with me, I'm fifty. Oh, the freedom of loving their maleness while not wanting to make them part of your economic unit.

And then there is you, about whom I was intending to write in the first place, before being diverted by these other matters. Looking at this embryonic new identity of mine I see it has very little to do with you. I have been your wife for so long. I have understood us and made us known to others as two. The cement was the sexual exclusiveness. From that mainstream arrangement a firm friendship has grown, fortunately for us, and for Jack.

Now that strict convention has been breached, it hardly seems to matter to the friendship. Though, having said that, I now have to say that I did weep yesterday morning. I woke with such a feeling — fear tempered with expectation. I said nothing but you turned to me and kissed me. Then we made love. It was good. I cried afterwards, a few big sobs. You hugged me and said my name over and over. "I'm not really sad, at least not all the time", I said. "I'm alright. It's just change, uncertainty, strangeness. I'm alright."

But I was talking about identity. And what I wanted to say will have to wait. Jack is at Ben's this weekend and you and I are going to see some all-American rubbish, the movie *Cliffhanger*. If it's only half as thrilling as *Raiders of the Lost Ark* (is that really over fifteen years old?), I'll be more than satisfied.

## Wednesday 25 August

Yes, *Cliffhanger* was aptly named. Amazing action. But why does every other word have to be fuck these days? And as for the lovingly-filmed violence, I closed my eyes. None of the irony, or the humour of *Raiders*, except for the very end when the gorilla Stallone has done away with the final villain and says, camera panning back until he's a dot hanging against the sheerest of sheer cliff-faces, "I'm outa here!" I laughed at that.

Last Saturday I had meant to write reams about my emergent identity as an independent woman. Then we went to the movies. Then Sunday happened. You and I lay talking in bed in the morning for three hours. I vowed to record all of it. So pivotal, it was. But now at least two-thirds of that conversation is out past Jupiter and climbing.

I remember the start. A quick cuddle before I got up and got on with some writing. The cuddle went on. And on. Then stroking. I'm thinking I'll get up at any minute. Then your erection. The stroking's fine, I think, but I don't want penetration. Do I tell you, I wonder. I just want to get up, really. Will that hurt your feelings?

You ask, "Do you want to make love?" Reading my thoughts. "No", I reply, "I want to get up and get on with things."

**You:** That's alright. I thought it better to ask. I was surprised last Friday when we made love. You'd said you wouldn't while I had a lover.

**Me:** I changed my mind—for then. I wanted to—then. I don't now.

**You:** That's fine. We've got to be honest about it.

**Me:** I know.

**You:** I won't tell you what's happening with me and this other relationship unless you ask; then I'll be honest.

**Me:** That's fine. So did you see her this week?

**You:** Yes.

**Me:** Both nights?

**You:** Yes.

**Me:** You're feeling OK about it?

**You:** Yes. It's really pleasant and enjoyable, and she seems to be much more "of the moment" than I am, not hassling for more time with me or anything like that.

**Me:** Is she a good person? Can you trust her?

**You:** I think so. She seems pretty honest. Nice sense of humour.

**Me:** Have you told her that I know?

**You:** Yes.

**Me:** What was her response?

**You:** She said, "Are you sure?", and I said, "There's the phone.

Give her a call". (*God, that is so like you. You can challenge the insides out of a person.*)

**Me:** Then what did she say?

**You:** She said, "Your wife must be a pretty special sort of person".

**Me:** What did you say to that?

**You:** I said, "Yes, she is *[aside]*, now get your gear off".

I knew from the look that the aside was for my benefit, to raise a laugh. And it worked.

Yes. Well. So it goes.

You're happier and I wouldn't say I was exactly unhappy.

You offered to get condoms, have them handy at home, in case of a repeat of last Friday. "Good idea", I said. "Make them good ones." Graham Chapman's Protestant in *The Meaning of Life* springs to mind again.

Margaret came to visit on Sunday. We talked marriage. We talked freedom. We are running on lines occasionally parallel. Good to have a friend who does not theorise, looks at things as they are when they are.

## Thursday 26 August

One memory of the conversation you and I had last Sunday morning has just returned. How could I have forgotten about it, when it was so startling to me? After affirming yet again that we were both happier with things in general than we had been in a long time, you asked if, at times when both Jack and I were away from home (which will be the case in the October school holidays), I would mind if you invited your girlfriend here, to our home.

I felt that same surge in my gut that I'd experienced when, back in April, you first said you wanted more separation in our marriage. That same surge I'd felt when you said yes, there were a couple of other women you were interested in, and then again when you said, a few weeks ago, you had finally had sex with one of them.

So. This one you now want to bring here, to my bed. I was amazed that you'd asked. Amazed that you'd think I would even consider saying yes. But I didn't react. I thought about my amazement for a while. I asked you didn't we agree that home was out of bounds? Yes, you said, but you had originally brought that up in reference to the possibility my having a lover here at home when Jack was around. You had not wanted that. And I had agreed. Not when Jack was around. But in the case of Jack not being around, you could see no objection to either of us entertaining our lovers here.

You were right about what we had agreed to. And your reasoning was sound. Reasoning always *seems* sound, being based on reason. My amazement *wasn't* based on reason. Just unadulterated honest emotion. And it was telling me, "So, here's another wedge between us, another nail in the coffin, another quantum leap towards total family anarchy, a defilement of my sacred site. How does he dare!"

So I said no in a very considered tone. I told you: "So far I haven't had a major problem with the rest of it, but I think I'd have a problem with that". You weren't insistent. But you were puzzled. You wanted to know what my reasoning was. But there was none. I didn't have reasons. Only feelings.

I began telling you which friends I had told about our saga. I hadn't talked to you about this before, but now I told you there were three: Margaret, Yvonne and Tricia. You didn't mind that. You were interested in their responses. Margaret and Yvonne have mostly just listened, and expressed admiration for the way we are dealing with it. Tricia's been the only one to react otherwise. And it was my remembering her words that brought us to this point in the conversation. Tricia asked me (and this was while your having another lover was still hypothetical), "If you and Noel were still having sex the way you always had, do you think he'd be doing this?" I said I didn't know, possibly not. Then she burst out, "That's what gets me about men! The premium they put on sex! When you've got such a good friendship, so much love, and they go ahead and break it all apart!"

I told you about this. I suppose I wanted to use it as an illustration of how intolerant many women are of the male sexual appetite. But not me. See the saint you have in me, Noel my darling. *I* don't think that way. *I'm* different. I agree with Germaine Greer when she says we like to think we've tamed sex by bonding the copulating couple in marriage, housed in a comfy nuclear unit for ever more. Bullshit we've tamed it. We've turned the male need to copulate into a monster that stalks city streets, that screams at us from every magazine stand and place of "entertainment", that is making our world a very dangerous place for women and children.

I told you all this, and I finished up, "So, you want more sex — go for it. But up the coast — not here". I was in the swing of it by now, and feeling generous, a smile on my face. And you laughed.

Well then, that was alright. We left it there.

And now! Several days later? I am looking at my response. Why do I not want her here? Friends and neighbours? There are no neighbours within view. The place is divinely secluded. Friends rarely visit without phoning, because of that seclusion. It's a bother to come out here and find that we're out. Keri sometimes ambles across the river. The chances of discovery are thin. But they exist. And I think of Jack. The story will out. And it mustn't happen that way. Not as "a story" from someone else, a rumour.

What else do I think of? This woman in *my* bed? Using *my* stove? Petting *my* Roger, the sacred cat? Playing with *my* Fred, the loopy dog? But would she make them any less mine? Can't I afford to share them? If she is the good person that you say she is, would she so defile them?

I, who have ranted against the folly of the nuclear family, who have known its dark corners ever since I was a child, will I now sit guarding this picture of my *own* narrow confines? Or can I let it expand, and embrace an image of Jack, my main worry, sitting down with you and me, and I am saying, "Dad's got a girlfriend. It's alright. We still love one another and are friends, and nobody's leaving anybody. But you might hear about or even meet Dad's girlfriend, so we thought it time to tell you".

Would such a move wipe away all my concerns? Would Jack's handling of it reflect our own? How civilised can we be? How idealogically sound? Do I now see myself greeting this woman as a friend, the second wife? Do I see myself as matriarch? Do I see with new eyes the family anarchy that I so feared last Sunday?

## Tuesday 31 August

A second part-time teaching job. At TAFE. Better paid, and the teaching just as rewarding. Growing financial independence. Growing excitement at the potential. And menstrual cramps.

## Thursday 2 September

A mean little bleed it was, creeping up on me after only nineteen days into my cycle and making my pre-menstrual back tell me, "You've gotta find a surgeon! You've had enough!" I thought I was back to square one again, after all my exercising and swimming and being good. Surgery, definitely. Then this silly little bleed. Oh is that all it's about. Just another early period. Two days. Then finish. Back feeling pretty good today. And a stimulating class too.

## Tuesday 7 September

I am lying low; very, very low. These last few days have seen me hanging in the gap, feeling the momentousness of almost any move I may make. It is not a happy time. Neither is it unhappy. It is a time for lying low, getting on with what needs to be done rather than what I want to do. What I *want* to do is to see the physiotherapist and other desirable men I know; go and flirt with them, be attractive to them, make them laugh with my incorrigible ways, but not invite them to my bed; not invite that complication.

Company. The company of men. I have always had it, always loved it. But my dear Grey and my dear Venky and Hugh are all in other countries, and my darling Al, who I laughed with on the subway, cried with at the movies, and cut capers with in the streets of Sydney, is dead of cancer. I want the company of men as friends, but I shall not seek it out. Not now. Not now while I feel so vulnerable.

I must be by myself now, and for a while. I must examine myself, my relationship to men, where the need I feel to hook a man is coming from.

I saw the physiotherapist again last week. Jack said it was time he went to him for a checkup, so we both went, I with my open mind and Jack, who likes the man enormously, with his innocence. It was good to see him and to speak to him free from the tyranny of infatuation. Afterwards, you were curious: was I still attracted to him? I told you I would welcome his friendship, but not as a lover. It was true at the time of speaking.

I also told you that I had been thinking about the coming holidays, when Jack and I will be in Sydney. I said you could bring your girlfriend here if you still wanted to. What's her name, anyway? Jan, you said. Okay. Her name's Jan. How old is she, anyway? She's forty-one.

Okay. She's forty-one. And she smokes. What? She smokes. But you *hate* smoking.

Well, I told you, I've been thinking about my initial response, and it was knee-jerk, it was fear, it was "what? have her here doing this with *my* things, *my* this and *my* that?" It was all *me, me, me* and *mine, mine, mine*. I saw that. I didn't like it. I'm nearly fifty for chrissake. It's time to break free of all that. What do I have to be afraid of? I can't see an answer to that question.

What I can see though is that you are a happier man than you've been in an age. Happier with me, happier with Jack, happier with Jack's friends. You and Jack are actually having fun together on the weekends. So as far as I'm concerned Jan is not a threat to my family. She may even become an extension of it.

You hugged me and hugged me and kissed me and kissed me. I felt shell-shocked. Shrapnel lodged in my brain. Was this me saying this? The sheer depth of these changes left me floundering there for a day or two, and I started thinking about all the lovely big men I know (they have to be big to be bigger than me). Thinking about how they look at me, smile at me, laugh at my jokes. Thinking how much I'd like to put my arms round them. Thinking, thinking, thinking.

I suppose seeing the physiotherapist again acted as a sort of catalyst. Even though I wasn't so attracted and it was much easier than last year, it still seemed to set off a train of thought, of longing. Longing for what? To be desired? Why? You desire me, you never stopped desiring me. Is that not enough? Why did I reject you? My libido's down. I'm menopausal. But if it's so down, what makes me capable of fantasising about other men? Am I still a gawky girl, gasping at Rhett Butler's audacity as he literally swept Scarlett off her feet? Am I still living in the land of the tinsel imagination?

Ai-yaah! as they say in New Guinea. Let's just put a lid on it for now. The path is muddy.

I am alone. Jack left this morning for nine days of camp. You will stay up the coast an extra night since Jack isn't home, making it three nights away. I could invite men here and throw myself at them. But no, no, no. I won't. I'll work instead. I'll write, prepare lessons, edit. I have a pile to do before the holidays, including a massive manuscript from the USA that I must turn around in ten or so days. I must make money. I am committed (by my own heart) to paying for the renovations to the barn and for the meditation sala. It's my vision, not yours. I must make money. I must stay quiet.

I am alone. I swim. I do yoga. I fast on Mondays. I juice fruit and vegetables each day and drink their goodness.

### Friday 10 September

It's 2.30 a.m. You just woke me up coming to bed, having fallen asleep in an armchair while reading *Real Magic* by Wayne Dwyer. I woke with a start, thinking, "There's somebody in the house!" It has happened a few times, on your first night back here. Obviously has something to do with getting used to you not being around. I know I won't get back to sleep without making some kind of movement first. The mind is too busy.

I am feeling very removed from you. So I have removed myself from you. And here I am. It was either sit and write or lie in bed crying. I've chosen to sit and write, and I know you are lying awake in the next room listening to the sounds of the keyboard.

I'd been looking forward to you coming home this evening and to having dinner with you. But you called to say you'd forgotten about the school meeting you had to attend. Did I want to have a snack with you at the beach cafe and perhaps attend the meeting too? No I didn't. Still feeling tired after a brandy-binge with Keri. Don't feel like going out. See you later.

Anger flaring from somewhere. Don't know where. Took the anger to bed. Now here I am, writing.

Feeling terribly bereft all of a sudden, and very teary. Nothing to do with being pre-menstrual either (though it's impossible to be certain in these days of hormonal gymnastics).

It is so beautiful here. I took the dog for a walk down to the river yesterday at sunset. I stood on the bank watching the stars arrive and the horses came to greet me, to see what treats I had, bumping me with soft noses. I had nothing to offer but they stayed anyway, letting me stroke their folded-felt ears. I love horses' ears.

I know little enough about the environment you live in while you're up the coast, though I've met one or two of the peole you work with and call friends. I am mystified: why would a person not want to come home to this beautiful place whenever he could? Is freedom from me so very attractive?

I feel bitter tonight. Still hanging, but bitterly, unhappily. I acknowledge the unhappiness, but I don't want to share it with you tonight. I want to stay closed up. I remind myself of what I said to you a while ago—that my struggle over what I feel about these changes is not over yet. Perhaps this has been brought on by your decision to stay up there an extra night this week and to return there a day earlier—next Sunday instead of the usual Monday. Because Jack is away, so you don't have to be here for him. And I find myself thinking, "So he really is only coming back for Jack; I'm not in the running". Silly, self-serving, self-pitying sentiments. I do myself and you an injustice. I know you love me, are my dear friend. But still I feel this gap in my heart. If you walked in now I don't think I could bear to meet your eye.

Keri dropped in early Tuesday evening with the finest bunch of flowers for me — roses and freesias and lots more. Heady stuff. I've been carrying them around in their vase, positioning them beside the computer as I write, on the desk as I edit, by the bed as I sleep. Such perfumes.

She doesn't often drop in unannounced, and I liked her timing. I had just poured myself a brandy and crème de cacao on ice and was settling down for a read. "Just a short visit. The flowers are to say thanks for looking after the animals while I was away." At midnight, three brandies and half a bottle of wine (and mercifully a healthy snack) later, she fled declaring, "I still haven't locked away the chooks!"

We'd spent six hours talking about our personal lives in the way that I suspect only women can. She was shattered by the news of your girlfriend. "I thought you were the perfect couple ..." "Perhaps we are", I said, "by not being in one another's pockets". I meant it then, but I doubt I would offer such a suggestion in my present mood.

But the irony of sharing all this with Keri. After all, it was she who stirred up feelings of jealousy in me not *that* long ago, vis-a-vis her hail-fellow friendship with you. I had thought I was the only one around that could relate to men in such a chummy way.

And look at us now. We turn out to be friends — her own marriage has its quiet problems — and indeed we declared our friendship over I think the second brandy.

The ambivalence about alcohol is with me still. That's twice in the last three weeks I've drunk more than I should, regretting it bitterly the following day. Though I still went for my early morning swim. I stood in the shower afterwards and suddenly brought to mind my meditation practice and how thoroughly I have lost my mindfulness in these last several weeks. I sit almost every day, but I am not engaged in it. It is habit. A habit I'll maintain. Mindfulness will return. It will.

In the meantime, your meditation practice snowballs. I taught you the basic metta technique last weekend, and you said yesterday you'd like to discuss it further in the next day or two.

Good thing I've got a sense of humour.

## Tuesday 14 September

Well I went back to bed after writing that last entry and slept till about 7 a.m. You'd already had your sit by the time I got up. You wanted to talk. I knew last Wednesday's phone conversation was weighing on you, when I'd shared with you my feelings about wanting the company of men, wanting to be attractive to them and so on, while at the same time recognising the need to lie low, to be quiet, circumspect.

You harped on the "other men" part, wanting to know how seriously I was considering having an affair. More anger, but directed at you this time. "For God's sake get off it!" I said. "Do you think that's the only possible way I can bridge this chasm in my life!"

As I write this now I am thinking, what chasm was I talking about? It seems to have clean disappeared. Remarkable thing, the mind.

So. Perhaps some cobwebs were blown away by all that. You were concerned about my seeing the physiotherapist again. I reiterated my lack of sexual interest. When we were out for dinner the following evening (Saturday) you were big enough to admit that, in your present state, you would find it very difficult to cope with my having another sexual partner. Told you that you needn't concern yourself about it, in your present state.

Talked too about the balance of your life. Much love for me and gratitude to me expressed. "You're not always pleasant to be with", you said, "because you challenge me. Jan is easier to be with. But I need your challenge. I need that."

It's raining. The young trees are jumping. Jack comes home from camp tomorrow. I've been working very hard, teaching and editing.

## Wednesday 15 September

Great excitement from Jack. The camp was a resounding success. A dingo ate half his school bag and bit into his plastic lunch-box. The bag now jettisoned. The lunch-box with gnawed corner, by contrast, an icon.

## Wednesday 29 September

I'm at Chittaprabha's place in Sydney. Eating banana toast. Thinking about how long it is since I wrote in my journal. And not caring much, really.

Chittaprabha and I have been talking, talking, talking. I can't describe fully the anchorage she provides for me; I know it's there, that's what counts. Her years of meditation and commitment to the dharma have given her a rare kind of surety. I look at her and I smile at that. I bathe in it. It is a kind of haven. I have seen some other friends, found a welcome everywhere. But hers were the only eyebrows that didn't shoot up at my news of you and your girlfriend, of our being "unmarried".

I spoke to you on Sunday morning. I phoned from the Elliots' place, where Jack is staying. As you had told me she might, Jan had joined you at our home on Saturday night, after Jack and I had left on the overnight bus. She'd met the dog, the cats, taken the walk down to the river. And, I assume, slept in my bed.

I felt very little at this news, very little. Just a sense of

"Well, that's what's happening"; a sense of the "suchness" of things, as Buddhists say. What *should* I have felt and by whose criteria? You sounded fine. In the room next to me I could hear Jack and Andrew playing a computer game. I had two weeks of talking, walking and meditation ahead of me. I was fine too.

## Thursday 30 September

Woke this morning from a dream of jealousy, in which I screamed at you after you'd informed me you'd be spending more time up the coast because "Uncle Noel" was in great demand by the "children"—whose I don't know. What about Jack, I screamed, etc., etc. Rotten dream. Glad to come out of it.

I did some early-morning yoga and was feeling good. Then you phoned, about 7.30 a.m. How was I! Fine. So were you. And all the animals. You were still at home. You hadn't gone up the coast to work. Had bent the rules, such as they are, around a few local clients. Jan was still with you at home. She had a week's holiday. How convenient, I thought. And none of this planned before I went away? It certainly wasn't mentioned.

Then you volunteered, "But there's nothing for you to worry about, nothing at all". I wondered what you meant.

I felt remarkably OKAY. I said to you, "I'm not worried, though I couldn't tell you why". I told you about the dream; how there may be unconscious worries; how my sits had been harmonious, revealing nothing but an intangible contentment.

I wonder—am I a fool?

Hard to answer that.

But one thing I see that interests me: yesterday, the twenty-ninth of September, Pluto was at 23 degrees 38 minutes of Scorpio, its third and final square to my natal Venus. As from now the symbol of death and rebirth will leave my personal relationships alone for quite some years. Meanwhile retrograde Saturn moves into the conjunction with my Venus, becoming absolutely and thoroughly exact on the twenty-fourth of October, at 23 degrees 38 minutes of Aquarius, where it then goes direct and so sits on that very point for eight days. Rarely do I look ahead in this way, knowing as I do the power of self-fulfilling prophecy. But, really, the symbolism fair drips from this one, and I am *fascinated*: " ... Relationships that have no purpose or that have outlived their purpose in your life will be cut off. Often you will be reluctant to let go of them ... "

## Friday 1 October

This morning's meditation chock-a-block with thoughts of sex, fantasising about some of the sweet, sweet men I know.

Chittaprabha and I ate out last night. A delicious Thai meal at my favourite spot, but still we found it hard to get off the subject of men and really into the food. Does the sex-thing never end? Will we be rocking and rolling with sweaty abandon in our dreams when we're ninety? We talked about ageing, our ageing; and sexuality, our sexuality. How one seeks sexual love because it seems to be the only way to really get close to another being. Sad, eh? Because it doesn't last, and we're conditioned to want what's good to last.

We also talked about lesbians, which we are not. Supreme disinterest. We like men.

## Saturday 2 October

Here again on retreat among the eucalypts, scene of my first retreat. (When Chittaprabha asked me what I was expecting and I said a holiday and she said, "It's better than a holiday", and my oath she was right.) Scene of my return to poetry, my return home to the dharma. Many memories. But no nostalgia. Only that centredness held by the sounds of birds, of rain in the trees, and glimpses of deep friendship.

Driving here yesterday, Chittaprabha and I talked of the parallels in our lives; her own lost but loving marriage. You are with Jan these two weeks, but I feel no jealousy. No fear. Yet I feel I am in mourning. I told Chittaprabha I didn't know what I was mourning.

"It's change", she said. "You're mourning the change."

Yes, that's it. Exactly.

And even though I know this change must happen if any of us is to find further growth and richness, still I look upon its happening with sadness. Because the change came, as change generally does, out of necessity rather than real understanding. It was you who kicked it off by saying you couldn't go on the way we had been. Your saying that gave me some courage. The fact of your saying it shifted my mind-set sufficiently for me to consider the necessity for ACTION.

In an almost two-hour sit this morning the plane of my consciousness grew vast, until it was all that there was. A horizon of light, warmth, safety. Infinite connectedness. Infinite joy. Then you put your hand on the raw spot at my back, invoking light and space in the place of pain.

## Monday 4 October

Two things about myself: first, what is traditional, what is accepted by others as conventional wisdom, seems to mean very little to me. My direct experience is all that I wish to cite. This is enormously liberating. And second, in a state of expanded consciousness I may experience the space around any phenomenon, observing it and acknowledging the "suchness" of it. Not reacting to it. I carried this experience of "space" into ordinary daily life when I was a child, though then it was unconscious. I carry it with me still, though in certain situations I have to bring it about consciously. At this point on my path, changing myself must be an act of will. Later, perhaps, the more "awake" me will be less conscious of her need to construct spaces around phenomena. She will see the spaces and the interconnectedness, as she did in childhood, as a matter of course.

## Wednesday 6 October

Still at Chittaprabha's. Returned from the short retreat on Monday. Continuing doing a lot of meditation, and seeing various friends, mostly dharma friends. Today I saw Julie. What a treat. She has resigned from the high-profile well-paid job she's held for twenty years, effective from January. She will let her house, live on the rent, move into a communal home with two or three other Buddhist women friends, and do voluntary hospice work. She was aglow. And I caught some of it. I think her age is relevant. She's nearly fifty.

Tomorrow is zoo day. I take Jack and Andrew to Taronga Zoo, and give Andrew's mum a break. Bet the first port of call will be the reptile house.

You phoned yesterday morning. You sounded well.

## Thursday 7 October

I woke with a feeling of expansiveness, that almost physical feeling I had while on retreat, mostly when I was meditating but sometimes not. My body as two open doors; light pours out. Whatever may wish to assail me can only pass through the doors and be touched or not touched by the light, as the case may be. It cannot stay with me. I cannot take it inside me. I am not vulnerable to it. With the doors open

I am supremely invulnerable. If once I close the doors the assailants can bump up against them, can knock me down. And I will react in kind.

The assailant treats me as though I'm worthless. If I already believe I'm worthless, with the doors closed against my own light, their treatment will have its desired effect upon me. I'll agree with them that I'm worthless. I'll react "badly", show them they're right. And so it will go on in a self-perpetuating downward spiral.

But if my doors are open, if I see and know my own light, let it shine out, I'll not take in their effort to turn me against myself. I will remain at peace with myself, and respond with some degree of compassion to my assailant's own suffering. Perhaps not at first, but maybe after a while, my peaceful responses will in some small way begin to change their behaviour towards me. And the spiral turns upward.

I'm in love with the open doors.

And I'm reminded of something in the Buddhist Pali Canon:

*It rains right through the thatch,*
*It rains not through the open.*
*So open up the thatch,*
*Thus it will not rain through.*


### Saturday 9 October

You phoned yesterday afternoon. A long and loving conversation. Jan is with you again at home this weekend. I am alright. You are alright. Though sadness comes and goes for us both. You said, "I've told her Jack is my priority. She understands that. So far it's alright. Whether it'll continue to be alright, who knows?"

Jack had his arm around me a lot the other day as

we wound our way around the zoo. And him with a friend in tow, too! Such a display of fondness touched me. We had fun. And it *was* the reptiles first. The Gabon viper had put on a few kilos since we last saw it. I fell in love with the bobcat ("Are you *still* looking at him, Mum? Come on. If I win a million dollars I'll buy him for you"), and I went to the sponsorship cottage to give some money. "I'm in love with the bobcat", I said, "and must sponsor it." But it was $50.00. My face fell. "You get a free pass", she said. "But I don't live in Sydney." Then she told me the sponsorship money all goes into a pool anyway, for all the animals. "Otherwise the reptiles would never get anything", she added. Well, my money was for the bobcat alone. But I couldn't afford $50.00. She wished us a nice day anyway.

I paid homage again to the amazing snow leopards. It says in Kipling's *Jungle Book* (I think) that animals cannot look for long into the eyes of humans. Not so with snow leopards. They seem to know your soul.

Dinner with Bill last night. One of our oldest and dearest friends in Australia. He listened and he offered me his love. He, who I've admired so long for turning around his entire life when he was past fifty, leaving behind the "hod carrying" that was his legacy from working-class Manchester and giving himself full-time to his crusade for social justice. "I've always loved you", he said, "ever since you walked into that first peace-group meeting and started talking, I've loved you. It wasn't sex, but I suppose I always thought that Noel would take it amiss if I'd told you that if ever you needed me, I'd be there. That's how conventional I can be. But I'll say it now. I'd be there."

I hang onto such words, despite my bid for "freedom". I see how dear to me my male "protectors" are. With Bill how can one feel anything but safe? There are tears in my eyes now. I know I'm pre-menstrual, but I'll still let these feelings happen and I'll still write them down. Right now I'm not so sure that I can cope without the physical presence and the strength of a man, a big, beautiful man, a man like you, or Bill, or Hugh—who has known my vulnerability since we worked together twenty-five years ago and whose love all the way from England still feeds me. Why do I need to belong? Why am I not bigger than that?

### Monday 11 October

The last two days with the Elliots. And, in this past two weeks of baring my soul to old friends, who should move me most deeply with his response but the arch-cynic Gareth. Seeing Jack and me off on the bus yesterday he hugged me like he's never hugged me before and said, "I love you, hmm? Give us a call soon. And not just a social chat. I love you". His kids looked bemused. Dad? What?

No sexual allusion here. I'm twice the guy's height for starters. Jack is only four inches short of the top of his head. Little Gareth, guaranteed to expose the blackest side of any given situation, who will pin out your mind on a dissecting board before changing to that characteristic "Anyhow, have a Winfield" levity.

Well, I was proud. You have to earn love from one such as he.

And so home. An overnight bus ride, pick up the car in town, stop for bread and milk and bump into you, stopping on your way up the coast to say hello to us. Both pleased and not pleased to see you. Gave you a hug, got one back. Not feeling much. Jack: "Hi Dad", from the passenger seat. Tired kid. Didn't get out for a hug.

**You:** Good holiday?

**Jack:** Yep. (*Why are my expectations higher? See you Wednesday evening. 'Bye.*)

Home. Things in reasonable order. But tall weeds between the citrus trees. Grass needs cutting. He's not been doing much work around here these last three weekends, that's for sure.

They've enjoyed a few bottles of white wine, I see. And shit, they could have emptied the waste bin in the bathroom.

Otherwise nothing. Only a sadness. My word, such a sense of loss. I walk down to the plantings with the excited dog lolloping behind me. So many weeds around the new trees. You phone from work. I can't talk to you easily. "I'm depressed", I admit, "so many weeds. So much work to do." But I think that is not the real reason. You phone again later, to see if I'm feeling any better. I guess you love me. But today I'm not sure what to do with your love. Is that because I have no label for it?

### Friday 15 October

On Wednesday night you came home with flowers. They were lovely. But I wasn't impressed. I sit here now looking at the cobwebs in the study window and I get a picture of how couples keep house on their dreams of togetherness. Houses! Who was it that called them brick trees for humans? Homes for humans, built by humans to withstand change, something the humans themselves can't do.

I've been thinking about the poem I wrote to you a long while ago, while I was on a meditation retreat. I called it "Coming Home":

> *If I come to you as one whose castle is built upon the movement of time*

*As one who knows only Change, which has no abode*

*If I come to you with a heart prepared for anything,*
*Open to the vagaries of the market and the lack of a full*
*freezer*

*If I come to you as one to whom the forward-plan of modern*
*life*
*Is an arid plain of profit and loss, an endless horizon of*
*hunger*

*If I come as one distressed at nothing but the wounds people*
*inflict,*
*Fearing nothing but the hatred in my own heart,*
*As one who hears above the daily din of greed*
*The ancient song of the trees, and knows that it is good*

*If I come to you no longer a little bit of a human being,*
*Will you — who are so fine and strong and capable —*
*Will you look into my eyes?*
*Will you let me in?*

You read it once. Put it aside. Never referred to it again.

Everyone thinks I'm so much happier than I really am. That's because I can't bring myself to say how much I'm hurting. I know it'll pass. So I leave it. Why bother people with clouds in transit? I tell them I'm well. Even if Chittaprabha herself were here with me now, though I'd tell her my mind, I would probably decline to cry on her shoulder.

I think my meditation is helping me gain this space between myself and my grief. It is a matter for me and my cushion, so to speak. As I sit each morning I feel complete. My zafu symbolises the wholeness.

So dinner on Wednesday night was a strain. You knew I wasn't relaxed. Wasn't happy to see you. Was preoccupied. For some reason you picked me up on semantics a few times. The final parry was when I said to Jack, "A lot of parents can't tell their children, 'No'", talking in general terms about lack of discipline. "They *choose* not to", you interjected, in what I think of as your lecturing tone. "It's all a matter of choice." It annoyed me. "I realise it's a matter of choice", I said, "I think I know something about choice."

"Stop arguing", said Jack. He is sensing the change. I know he is. "We're not arguing", you said. "Yes we are", I said, "Jack is right." I winked at Jack to soften the mood and continued to argue my point. Later I asked myself why I'd laboured at it, why I'd been so ratty, as if I didn't know I was pre-menstrual.

I said to you after Jack was asleep, "I'm feeling estranged from you, more than ever, just in case you were wondering. I'm trying to keep up appearances for Jack's sake, but it's hard. Hard to be even civil. I'm going to bed. Are you planning to sleep in the same bed?"

You looked hurt, confused. I didn't care. Then you shrugged. It was defensive. "Whatever you like", you said. So I told you, "You decide, whatever's appropriate. Goodnight".

I dreamed about Sangharakshita, the founder of the Western Buddhist Order. He was coming here (and it really looked like here) to visit us (you and me) and I was feeling elated. When he arrived at the gate of the house paddock I saw to my dismay that there were several other visitors, not connected with him, arriving at the same time. They were all old friends and acquaintances with whom I felt I no longer had much in common. But I still had to greet them and be polite. I was torn. They swarmed around us. Sangharakshita came up to us and said something like, "Now let's see what kind of people you are". He circled the two of us and said, "Yes, quite normal". I was for some reason pleased by this, and also had a fleeting thought about you wanting to be included in what (I think) was to be a bid for a deeper commitment to Buddhism. All the other visitors had gone on into the house, looking a bit put out by the amount of attention we were giving to the strange English monk with the hybrid accent. More feelings of discomfiture on my part.

I woke thinking the symbolism of that one was more than obvious. Got up at 5.30 a.m. for a sit and then a swim, but the bleed started as soon as I was upright. Oh yes, that again. I had an hour's sit. The bleeding put paid to the swim. Never again will I swim while wearing a tampon. Three vaginal infections have taught me that.

You had your sit. You hugged me hard before driving off with Jack to the school bus and then to work.

Yesterday's writing class, the first of this term, was a bottler. An inspirational group. I smiled when one of the older ones asked Christie how she could write so brilliantly about things she couldn't possibly have experienced. "You're so young", she said. Ah, yes, but the young are born with their own wisdom aren't they? And some of them, like Christie, have clearly been here more than a few times before.

Last night I cooked dinner. And the night before. But I have lost interest in feeding you. There was a time when it gave me pleasure, but no more. I begin to associate the modern kitchen with a new form of female bondage.

I've been thinking about the barn. When the renovation is done and it's habitable, why don't *I* move in there? All I ever wanted was a simple place to live, surrounded by green and trees and water. I didn't want a multi-bedroomed suburban home to keep clean and tidy, but that's what marriage to you handed me.

You could have the house. You could keep it clean. You could spend the time moving your effects from point A to point B. You could have your girlfriend here. You would, I'm sure, be kind enough to guarantee me peace and quiet, since the barn is quite close to the house, when and if I have fellow meditators here for retreats. I could still build my sala in the forest remnant, when the money permits. And I could ask Ron to work on the stable for extra sleeping space for retreatants. That way we won't have to bother you at all.

I would put my earnings in a separate bank account and just live on that. I would only ask you for cash for Jack's needs. I'd rather like that. Jack could commute as he wished between the two dwellings. You would have no more jurisdiction over me nor I over you. This would be a co-operative and harmonious way of maintaining a bond of friendship for our own sakes, as well as our son's.

Yes, I can see it all.

And it's been brought on by the realisation of my own weakness in the years you and I have been together. You're not a domineering person, but you're impressive, with that air of being sure of yourself and your rightful position in the status quo, which you basically endorse. The tiny light of rebellion that shone in you when we met wasn't fanned by my quiet outrage at the grab-too-much system. It was extinguished. "Buy a house!" I said. "What for? We're going to Australia, remember?" But we bought. And we profited. Came here. Bought and profited again. And you worked, played games with money that I don't understand. Made us comfortable.

Finally came the resentment. Not voiced, but implied, quietly. It's been eating away for years. Why wasn't I playing the game too? I didn't seem to be interested. Yet I benefited from it. Oh, I earned some money. I've always earned a little bit—paid for the endeavours that were ephemerally and exclusively mine. But accumulation has been your bag.

Perhaps it's time to let you have the accumulation in its entirety and for me to cease all pretence and distance myself (a little way, as far as the barn) with all that I need.

My clothes. A word processor. Some books. Pens and paper. My meditation cushion. A phone, yes, I'd have to get a phone hooked up. I doubt I'd need a fridge. And definitely no TV. The cat's dishes. They'd be over in a flash.

You just phoned. You wanted to talk. I still don't feel like talking, especially not over the phone. Told you later, maybe. Maybe tonight.

The timing of this my homecoming could have been better. Coming back to little evidences of your recently-estranged husband's lover when you're forty-nine and pre-menstrual is a tall order indeed.

## Monday 18 October

I've just looked at the beginning of this journal. I see that I began it on the first of November. Almost a year ago. I still have not re-read any of it. But I shall soon. I'll read the whole of it. As soon it is a year old I'll make myself a cuppa, sit down with it and review the year's events and non-events. No doubt I'll laugh. And cry.

More changes.

Driving home from the beach yesterday you took my hand and squeezed it just as I was about to do the same to you. So I squeezed back. I love you for the life that has for years flowed through you to me. You are inextricably a part of me.

It is the talking that opens the doors, opens the hearts. I sat in the sand looking out on the ocean and listed for you the disappointments of my homecoming. The thought-lessness of things left lying about. You apologised. Offered no defence. I know from years of slightly amazed observation that you do not see the same as I do. For example, you are incapable of noticing dust on things.

We talked of our old friends, their responses, of your growing attachment to Jan, my growing attachment to freedom. Of Jack. Of my moving into the barn ("If you did that, we should just tell Jack that we are following divergent paths, but that we're both still here for him. We shouldn't tell him 'Dad's got a girlfriend'. After all, I may not have a girlfriend tomorrow.") We talked about that too. Jan's apparent uncertainty about her relationship with her ex-husband. Will she/won't she have him back? You want your relationship with her to continue, but recognise it may end any moment.

We talked of sex. Again. Is it just sex? Nobody seems to know. "If what Margaret Mead called 'post-menopausal zest' strikes me and I start looking around for men again, do you think you'll regret not having maintained patience for a few years?"

You said, as one might expect, you didn't know. How could you? It's the kind of loopy hypothetical question I detest. But I couldn't stop myself from asking it. "My biggest fear is that I get left out in the cold on all fronts. You and Jack have gone your own ways and don't want to know me, and I'm hopping from relationship to relationship, which is not really my way, as you know."

Yes, I do know. That is not your way. Nor is it mine.

Later on, when we were lying down together for a rest (on our bed which Jan apparently would not go near, not even into our bedroom, and I thank her for that), you kissed me on the arm, said, "We have to help one another".

### Sunday 24 October

A busy week. Full of writing articles, preparing lessons. You came home Wednesday and dropped a remark about not having talked to your friend Louise for ages. So where have you been staying on Monday and Tuesday nights? You had told me you didn't stay for the whole night whenever you were at Jan's place.

So I asked if you had started sleeping over at her place?

Yes. Since when? For the last few weeks.
Then an outburst:

**Me:** Why didn't you tell me about the change!
**You:** Sorry, I thought I had.
**Me:** No, you hadn't. And I don't bloody like it. I don't like you
leaving me in a position where I might have phoned Louise to
talk to you, and then she would experience the embarrassment
of my obviously not knowing, and I would experience the
embarrassment of her embarrassment, and so on. Never
bloody do anything like that again, or the deal's off!
**You:** What deal?
**Me:** The deal about you being my "friend". You're not my friend
if you behave like that.
**You:** Sorry, sorry, sorry. I really did think I'd told you.
**Me:** Like hell you thought you'd told me! (*At which point you left
the room.*)


I went to bed. Before falling asleep I promised myself and
on Jack's behalf that I would not indulge in such an
outburst again. You had no reason for deliberately not
telling me. It was thoughtless, that's all, like your not
emptying the bathroom waste-bin earlier this month. You've
given me a pretty honest account of your feelings and
movements thus far.

I had to acknowledge my jealousy. How affronted I feel
because Jan is an office clerk — an office clerk! And I had
to acknowledge what I have sensed in you this last week
or so, that you are only half here; that you're falling in
love (oh, perish the term!); that you'd much rather be with
Jan all the time.

So. All this I acknowledged. To myself. And the following
morning to you. Said sorry for the outburst. Told you my
thoughts. Yes, I'm jealous. Not that you're in a nice sexual
relationship and I want one too. Not that. I don't want

one, not now, not yet, not while I'm still struggling from the egg.

**You:** What is jealousy?

**Me:** Holding on. Clinging. It's fear. The fearful and jealous part of me wants to hold onto you because it's afraid of the unknown, the bizarre possibility of facing life without you. And that's what I feel in my lowest moments. That and outrage. Outrage that you've left me for an office clerk! These are my thoughts. I'm not asking you to respond or give me answers, I'm telling you what's going through my head. I'm looking at you and thinking, what have all our years together been about, all that creative energy, that special relationship that our friends sensed and envied, if you up and leave me for an OFFICE CLERK!

**You:** I haven't left you. If I'd left you I wouldn't be here now.

**Me:** Yeah, yeah, yeah. I know that. But my mind is choked with clichés right now and I'm working my way through them. It's a matter of time. As with all the other changes, I need time to accommodate this one, and accommodate it creatively, not by thinking in dead-end terms like "having an affair", "in love with someone else", "leaving me for a clerk" and the like. I need time. In that time there may be other outbursts. I'm trying though. I'm trying.

In my best moments, when my "doors" are open, I see there's no blame. There's only the busy-ness of Change, how what we each have to offer has moved and shifted and sometimes pounded against the shoreline of our expectation over the years. How we inflict pain upon ourselves by not acknowledging those waves, grinning foolishly as they break against our social-sexual-cultural-faces. Well, I want to surf those breakers rather than try to stop them.

You didn't deny it when I said I could see you'd "fallen in love", that you'd prefer not to have the responsibility of us. You just reiterated that you hadn't left us; that you'd assured Jan your priority was Jack.

(Comic relief: I just heard Jack warning his friend Ben about my herbal tea that's in the glass jug: "Don't drink that! It's rough. It's disgusting. It's Mum's. And it's expensive".)

You're working hard this weekend—lots to do outside. Me too. In my garden all day yesterday. Surrounded by life. And the noise of kids having fun together.

I told you this morning that while I still expect further tears, I think in the end it will be alright. Just as I've always thought, ever since childhood. Things with me will be "alright" because I feel basically "alright" about myself. That feeling of "alrightness" that has annoyed you so often, Noel, over the years we've been together. My she'll-be-right approach. What was it Robyn Davidson said about that? The closest thing to a Zen statement ever to come out of Australia?

And you said yes. It's only now that you'd come to understand it too.

## Wednesday 27 October

I am feeling so assaulted by the world that I have almost become a spectator of my own assault. This helps to distance me from total self-pity. I wrestle with sentences to describe my alienation, but I cannot pin them entirely to the ground. Parts of them continue to thrash about and nip at me from behind.

Saturn is astride my natal Venus this very week. My neck is tense. My neck is *never* tense. But this week, my neck is TENSE. I work. I lie low. I look for signs.

Yesterday, flicking through an ancient book recently lent to me by a 94-year-old gentleman friend, a bookmark, brown at the edges, fell out. It bore the famous words from

1 Corinthians 13 that I had not read in many years, the Good News Bible translation:

> *I may be able to speak the languages of men and even of angels, but if I have no love, my speech is no more than a noisy gong or a clanging bell. I may have the gift of inspired preaching; I may have all knowledge and understand all secrets; I may have all the faith needed to move mountains — but if I have no love, I am nothing. I may give away everything I have, and even give up my body to be burned — but if I have no love, this does me no good.*
>
> *Love is patient and kind; it is not jealous or conceited or proud; love is not ill-mannered or selfish or irritable; love does not keep a record of wrongs; love is not happy with evil, but is happy with the truth. Love never gives up; and its faith, hope and patience never fail.*
>
> *Love is eternal. There are inspired messages, but they are temporary; there are gifts of speaking in strange tongues, but they will cease; there is knowledge, but it will pass.* For our gifts of knowledge and of inspired messages are only partial [my emphasis]; *but when what is perfect comes, then what is partial will disappear.*

## Thursday 28 October

This is hard. This is very hard. I cannot remember ever feeling this afraid, this alone. And yet I want to maintain that aloneness. I need it at this time. It scares me and it hurts me, but I need it. I need to sit, to think, to wait, to watch, to attend to my own heart. And when that process is over — I hope it will be soon — I will know better. And I will not be so afraid.

But it is hard. I want to share with my friends and I can't, because of Jack. I want to tell everybody that you and I are no longer married, that we are leading increasingly separate lives, that I am more and more on my own, and if they want to phone me and ask me to a movie or out to dinner or whatever then I'd be pleased. But they think we're still a couple when we're not. All I can do about this is sit and wait and watch.

You are seeing an old Sydney friend this evening, up the coast, and won't be home till late. Jack is sleeping over at a schoolfriend's as I am running an evening class. You told me you'd probably go back up the coast on the weekend as Jack won't be home. He'll be at Ben's for a big Halloween do. So I'll be on my own. A further chance for meditation and writing. To quietly sit out the slow movement of Saturn away from my Venus. And then ... ?

## Friday 29 October

Oh double bliss, oh triple joy! I got up, had a sit, hung out the wash, saw you and Jack off, came inside, went to the toilet—blood on the knickers! My period! This explains why I've been feeling it's The End Of All Things for the last few days. Furthermore, I've had almost nil pre-menstrual back pain this time, perhaps an indication that my back is well and truly on the mend. Furthermore again, this is only day sixteen of the cycle. More evidence of erratic periods! Menopause, here I come. Mind you, some women have erratic periods for years before actually having the menopause. But I refuse to consider that on this glorious morning.

I'm planning to spend the weekend in meditation while you are both away.

## Saturday 30 October

No menstrual cramps. Very dark bleed, and very little of it. Only one day's worth, really. I went for a swim this morning.

## Wednesday 3 November

I've just realised I let the anniversary of the opening of this journal, the first of November, pass without comment. Ah me. I was going to sit down and read it through for the first time, wasn't I? Forgot all about that. The first was a Monday. A day of flat tyres, flatter batteries, and cancelled classes.

It's only the second time I've had to change a wheel in seventeen years. So that took up most of my remembering. Little and big things going wrong add to the state of siege I'm currently experiencing, though my 24-hour meditation intensive on the weekend helped me along that fork in the road that is the present moment, and leads to the real world rather than the one I'd rather be in, dreaming about the ideal.

I stayed with myself and it seems I'm still here. I'm thinking about you a lot too, in terms of what you are and not what I want you to be. There have been some unpleasant self-pitying moments these last few weeks. I've just been sitting with them till they pass. Feeling basically calm.

## Tuesday 9 November

This journal has become onerous. I don't want to sit here doing this. But I feel I have to. Have to record some words. Keep the record up to date. Lest we forget. Oh dear. What a bore. There is far too much for me to ever get it right. I could well look back on these words in years to come and say to myself, "No, no, no, it wasn't like that at all".

So. What's happening today? How am I feeling at this very moment? Hungry. I'm fasting. I've made Tuesday my fasting day as I'm now teaching all day Monday. I've let the fasting days go by the board lately, since I've been doing more teaching. But a firm resolve has recently taken hold again, and Tuesday it is. As it's been a while since I did a serious twenty-four hours, I'm feeling it today. The pinched gut. But I'll stick it out. It'll be easier next week.

Had a blood test last week. Curious to see what if any deficiencies. Result: definitely menopausal, judging by hormone levels. A bit low in iron. Apart from that I'm the picture of health. Apparently alfalfa contains oestrogen (how strange) and prunes contain iron. The (male) doctor could tell me no more. I must consult the literature.

Generally though, certainly compared with this time last year, when I started this journal, I'm feeling stronger. More energy (not back to normal, but increasing), and much less back pain.

Spent a physically active weekend outside: gardening, tree-care, and—oh joy—swimming in the dam again. Jack and his friend Greg took the little dinghy down to the dam and found it virtually weed-free, good for boating and swimming. So you and I joined them.

You seem well. Our talks are quiet, searching, wanting to help rather than hinder. You give me hugs. Seem genuinely grateful for the understanding, tell me I'm amazing.

Am I? I love you and I love our son. That's all.

**Me:** Do you have a sense of loss?
**You:** Yes, I do. Of course I do.
**Me:** What was between us in our marriage was so special. Our friends all commented on it—do you miss that?

**You:** Yes. But the best chance we have of keeping what's always been special between us is in a non-nuclear situation.

While I would not say that my love or the warm domestic sex we have enjoyed over the last two or so years was particularly inadequate, I am reminded again and again of the powerful male drive to sow seed. Sobering newspaper headlines and delightful TV documentaries about various copulating creatures keep on bringing it home. So, how can this business of marriage possibly work?

It is not a realistic expectation. For myself, I have abandoned it. And I rejoice that I have, not a husband, but a father-of-my-child and a dear friend who was "man" enough to be honest about his need for increased copulation and a life and friends outside the home. Good on him.

Will it continue to work? No idea. We have a fighting chance. The foundation is strong.

We are still sleeping in the same bed. OK, it's a huge bed. Sometimes we cuddle, and it feels good, that continued intimacy. But as has been the case for a while now, I've no sexual desire for him. Whether he has for me I'm not sure. He said a few weeks back he was still getting used to not being my lover any more. We haven't discussed it since. I've not noticed any rampant erections lately.

Now I've always maintained it's possible for a couple to sleep in the same bed without having sex. But what concerns me is the continuing deception of Jack, who (I think) believes that nothing has changed. It bothers you too, I know. We would both prefer to be open with him about what's happening, but at the same time we are afraid of what his response might be.

This need to tell Jack, for my part, is a measure of the extent to which I am accepting the change. And sleeping in separate rooms cements that. In a sense I would almost feel obliged to sleep separately once Jack is told. Though you say it wouldn't bother you, our still sharing a bed. You say you like it. Though you would agree to separate rooms if a problem arose from sharing.

You've also said, more than once, that although you would like your relationship with Jan to continue, it could end any moment. She is ambivalent. Still trying to sort out other things in her life. A bit bemused by your continued closeness to me.

But you know, even if your new relationship did end, I doubt that you and I would "remarry".

Jack deserves to be told the whys of our separateness. Not the sex so much—I'm not sure how clear a picture a ten-year-old could have of that—but things like why we don't go away together on holidays the way we used to, and the fact that Dad spends time with friends up the coast when Jack is away.

It is the honesty that is important. We need to tell him: look, this has happened between us but it hasn't diminished our love and regard for one another, and our joy in being together with you.

When we were talking on the weekend about how best to "make it work"—how to cause the least amount of suffering to all concerned—I ventured, "The way it would work best is for me to become friends with Jan". You nodded.

I sketched a scenario: we tell Jack the reasons why we're no longer "married"; that is, the differences between us, wanting to pursue separate interests. Nothing about Jan. She came after the fact, which is of course true. And Jack should know she was not the cause. Then and only then we tell him about Jan, that I've met her, and am friends with her. It's cool.

It's possible that eventually you would visit Jan with Jack as well—who knows? But I wouldn't want to go into that with Jack at this stage. He'll need time to assimilate these new ideas.

You thought my scenario was very sound.

First question: meeting Jan. When and where? Answer: here. In a couple of weeks. Jack can go to Ben's.

I've looked at Jack's astrological transits, something I've never done before because I've long felt that a young child doesn't manifest them so strongly, and anyway, I have never wanted to see his life unfolding through any occult spectacles, until now. Now that he's hardening into a young person it's time to take the cosmic complexities into account. And the timing looks good, the most major thing happening for him in a few weeks being a Jupiter square to his Saturn, normally positive and potentially very growth-oriented.

Second question: will Jan *want* to meet me?

## Tuesday 9 November

Got an answer to my second question: yes, she's willing to meet, though feels odd about it (can't blame her), she's willing to do it "for the little fella". You phoned this afternoon to tell me that, and also to say hello, as you always do at least once whenever you're up the coast.

So there it is. I don't think I'm asking a third question.

## Saturday 13 November

I knew something was up when you came home Wednesday night. I wonder if it's that faculty that rams home the biggest nail of them all in the coffin of traditional marriage? The ability to read your partner like the proverbial book. Knowing that your partner is not as they seem; that inside they're discontent, puzzled, worried, seething. It's that intimate knowledge that spells a deprivation of privacy, even of one's own thoughts.

How refreshing not to be known! This is what makes meeting new people so exciting. One can start all over again, armed with the accumulating wisdom of years. For my own part, I'm coming to wonder to what extent I need such intimacy. And I see, too, that there are times when you would prefer my window into your mind to cloud over.

We didn't talk until Thursday evening, when I asked if you and Jan had agreed on a time for her visit. You said that two things had come up. (Here it comes, I thought.) First, she has family visiting over the next few weeks. Fine. Second, you've asked her to sort out her feelings for her ex-husband before you bring her further into our family picture.

You'd mentioned this complication before, quite a few times. But I hadn't realised to what extent it was an issue for you. You said you liked her "free spirit", as you called it in the first few weeks of the relationship. Perhaps you're now experiencing all the clinging tendencies that being "in love" implies.

I find myself wondering how Jan feels about *your* feelings for me, and our continued involvement. I didn't put that to you at the time. But I shall. Later today.

## Tuesday 16 November

You said that you and Jan haven't really talked about your still being "with" me. You reminded me that it's only been a relationship since August. You said Jan's ex wants her back, that much is definite, but that she doesn't know if she's still in love with him or not, and that if she does go back, it's possible that the ex might be doing you a favour.

We were walking through the paddocks, under the stars, Roger and Fred following, Roger yowling every two minutes, as he always does when he goes cross-country at night, telling us that he is right there behind us and not to let the bogey men get him. Love that cat.

You talking; halting, hesitant, confused — but honest. Never anything but honest.

Like me, you're at a significant crossroads in your life. You are treading very carefully. Demonstrating your concern for me, your concern for Jack. "If we do ever decide to be 'married' again", you said at one point, "we'll be stronger for this."

Later you asked me how I felt now about our move here from Sydney. I told you I felt good about the land, about my dream of making it available to the community to use for meditation, for horticulture, for reforestation, for whatever good purpose it lends itself. I said I felt that I was becoming part of a community for the first time in my peripatetic life — and such a community! So many creative people, people searching for, and living, alternatives to the mainstream madness.

For your part, you said you would never willingly return to Sydney or any big city, but the land has become "an irrelevance" for you. Having put so much energy into it in the first few years, you now have little left for it. You have told me you will help me in my endeavours with this place, and indeed I feel this is all you are doing now, letting me take the lead and make the decisions.

When we came here your vision was not shared by me. That I barely appreciated the work you did in putting up the cattle fencing and suburbanising the house paddock had its effect. While I was not critical, I was clearly not enthused. Why didn't we talk about this years ago? Because when you asked me if I would mind you keeping cattle and doing this and doing that, I was quite unaware of what these things entailed. And I didn't have the energy to argue. Dad had just died, my back was crippled, all my reserves had run dry. The years of you seeing me as an ingrate took their toll. You'd had enough of trying to please me, so you stepped back. And now you can see, I think, that I am, and always have been, on the level with my mad dreams of alternative ways.

Whatever the situation with Jan, you say you would still feel dissatisfied with your life, your lack of purpose. We talked about our respective upbringings. Me, working class; every step I took along the road to academia was greeted with gasps and praise. Mum said, "Never get married, darlin', it's 'orrible". Dad, in his gentlemanly way, was more circumspect, but the message was the same. You, WASP upper-middle class, parents "in the church"; the prison sentences of a university degree, marriage-ever-after and a beautiful home declared at birth.

You with great expectations. Me with none at all. These things have significance. In addition you are experiencing that "crisis of middle age" symbolised by its corresponding planetary transit—yes, folks, it's ... Neptune square Neptune, which, by the way, you have been labouring beneath since we moved here and which is now and only now moving off. Another retrospective victory for astrology—I only just took note of it in your chart this weekend as we talked. We looked it up together in *Planets in Transit*, and learned you were experiencing part of the "mid-life crisis" (I prefer "quest" to "crisis")—a time when you are likely to review your life and ask yourself probing questions about whether or not you have lived up to your ideals, achieved your goals. If you feel you have let yourself down, author Robert Hand says, there is a danger under the rather deluded Neptunian vibration that you may "go off half cocked"; following some kind of vision or ideal that is not worth following. You are advised to give yourself a long hard look, but not to act—yet. There is a warning against acting too quickly, which may lead to major disturbances; perhaps emotionally, perhaps domestically, perhaps professionally.

As with all astrological "predictions", nothing specific is "written", so to speak, except in the mind, and in the heart. Hand tells us that some of the insights that come to you during this time will be valid but others not so. In time, you will know which ones are which. In time.

Were the cattle the "half cocked idea"? When we moved here I remember thinking you'd expropriated my vision, diverted me yet again with your fences and your barbecues with other beer-drinking cattle types, of whom dear Keri was one, and by far the most pleasant, even if I was envious of her good looks.

I wanted to plant trees, to create a place of beauty, while the blood spurted from the de-horning of steers and the virtues of meat-with-every-meal were extolled by your new cockie chums. I had never disliked you before. But I disliked you then, quietly. You knew, though. Of course you knew.

And here, now, is where that knowledge has brought us. Just a few cows now, little heifers, no steers. You said last week you would only buy heifers in future, just for selling to breeders. No more steers to go off to the abattoir, in deference to my feelings.

I'm tired of writing about this. Lots of visitors lately. But I don't want to write about that either. I'm through.

## Monday 22 November

Day twenty-five of my menstrual cycle and not a smear in sight. Feeling last week as though it was about to start any minute, on the kind of short cycle I've been experiencing, then nothing. Felt physically well all weekend, during which I was quite active, planting new trees and fertilising established ones. There's still some movement going on down there, though—a phantom period? A non-starter? The menopause?

A good weekend together, doing and talking. On Friday

evening we came to what we think is a good decision about the bed business, which would be: First, the truth, and second, a lot less threatening than "Dad's got a girlfriend, but it's alright really", which is also of course the truth, but the meaning turns on the words you choose to express it, especially to a ten-year-old who dearly loves both his parents.

On Friday night, and Saturday night, and last night, I slept in the spare room, Dad's old room, and I'll continue to do so. Jack hasn't noticed. I get up so early anyway, before anyone else. But when he does notice and asks about it, as we imagine he will, this is the reply we thought would be the most skillful (to use a nice, precise Buddhist term): "Well, Dad's a noisy sleeper; he huffs and puffs and holds his breath and farts and sometimes I get jack of sleeping with him and find a bed somewhere else. The last time I did it I liked it so much I decided to keep on doing it. Dad doesn't mind. We don't have sex together any more and haven't for a long time, even though we still love one another very much, it's friends' love, not sex. So sleeping in different beds didn't seem to be a big deal."

Voila!

Sound good? Sound too much like theory? Is there a convolution waiting in the wings?

You were most definite that you didn't want Jan mentioned yet. Since you have your doubts about how much longer the relationship will last, I think you're probably right in this. A cynic might say it's guilt on your part. But I see your genuine concern for Jack. The introduction of a girlfriend who could dematerialise at any moment seems foolish. Of course she may not. In which case she will undoubtedly be introduced when appropriate. Along with any other girlfriends that may be deemed necessary—all at the appropriate times.

Whatever may happen regarding your sex life, for my

part I am feeling increasingly positive about the decisions we have made and are making. You occasionally refer to the idea that one day we may be married again, but I think you doubt it as much as I do.

And I don't miss the sex. No harm has come to me since I stopped. I don't feel I require therapy. And look at all the other places for that energy to go.

Having said that, I now remember how I felt last Friday when I was in town and bumped into Matthew. What a very attractive man, and thoughtful. Telling me that he's soon to move into a house of his own, and very close to where I live and how he wants to continue writing, and I cut in with "Oh you should join the next writing group I run, in February ..." without letting him finish what he was saying because I suddenly went all fluttery.

Talking to myself about it since then: "It would be nice to be friends. We have a lot in common. Even though he's physically devastating, I don't need to spoil it by thinking sex, do I? Sex has ruined many a good friendship. And shit, I'm nearly fifty and he's only forty-four. Why do I do this? Why can't I be attracted to someone older than me? Someone with grey hair, instead of latter-day hippies who stroke your arm and murmur, "Hey, nice talking to you".

He wrote down his phone number on a piece of paper and handed it to me. It's still in my wallet.

### Wednesday 24 November

Can't sleep. The class this evening was on a roll, they were brilliant. My mind's still running around in it. It, and you. You were home when I got back. Picked up Jack from James's place en route from work. You asked me what was "unfolding in my life at present". I didn't feel like talking and thought it a daft question. Felt very estranged from you. Almost antagonistic. Said very little. Cut my losses and went to bed in the spare room. Couldn't sleep. Here I am. Nearly midnight.

Feeling lonely. That "how can I cope without a man?" feeling again. Jack will be at Ben's all weekend and you will go up to Jan's for Friday and Saturday nights, rejoining us for dinner with Ben's parents Sunday evening. Looking at my beautiful land and seeing only the work there is to do. You called it an irrelevance in your life. How can I realise my dream to make this place available to the community? How can I have people here when I'm having to take into account this husband who is not a husband, when I feel I can't have Tom, Dick and Harry here helping to plant trees and make gardens and build buildings for free lunches and dinners and a doss without having your (the husband's) blessing. You won't want to come home from your sojourns up the coast and find the place turning into the communal something I want it to be.

But we must have people here. For me. For Jack. It is too hard and too lonely otherwise.

My period still hasn't started.


## Tuesday 30 November

You come home and do the wash, hang it out. Other jobs too. Ones you've done throughout our marriage whenever you've noticed they needed doing. Not for you "that's women's work". Nor for me "that's a man's job".

So many things have not changed.

You're not happy, seem burdened, all the time burdened. I broach the topic. "I don't think I've ever been what you'd call happy", you say. And I say, "You've never taken pleasure in little things, simple things". You agree.

I tell you how I enjoyed a meal I cooked for myself when I was on my own. You ask, "How do you feel, being alone?" I say, "Content. Not full of joy. I think I need to be with people for happiness. To know that some com-munication's going on gives me happiness. But I also know that it's a fleeting thing. When I'm on my own I'm content. So different from when I was young and only knowing how to define myself alongside other people. Seeking them out, to the extent of playing games with them, presenting myself this way and that way. Now I don't fear being alone. It's quietness inside. Easy. I need it. Though I wouldn't want it all the time. Not yet. Maybe when I'm eighty."

You tell me that Jan's ex-husband phones her up in the middle of the night when you are there to tell her he can't go on without her. She keeps getting upset about it. You say it's getting tedious and that if it continues your relationship with Jan will have to end. "That bad?" I ask. Yes.

"You can be independent of women, you know." I see that you don't know. You mumble a bit. I leave it.

We decided to do a nice easy resort holiday at the end of January. We've done nothing like that in ages and we thought it would be greatly appreciated by Jack. We'll take Ben along too.

Then your Dad rang to say he was coming to Australia for three weeks at the end of January. Dear George. The wheelbarrow's still recovering from the workout he gave it last year. Nearly eighty and he hardly let up on the farmwork once.

**You:** What will we tell him? Shall I write to him first and tell him about our being "unmarried"?

**Me:** No. Let him come and see us together. He'll see we are friends. Then we tell him. Same approach we're using with Jack—we tell Jack we've been "unmarried" for a while, and he realises we've still been friends in that time. It's good psychology, eh?

**You:** Yes.

Am I making this sound too easy?

Last night Jack and I walked along the riverbank under a full moon and saw the platypus again. Jack had his arm around me for the whole walk, talking, making sure I didn't step in any cow pats. I wondered what I'd done to gain entry to Utopia for fully half an hour.

Mothers and sons! Would I be at such pains to set things right with you if it were not for love of my son? I suspect that most mothers, like myself, do not think of it in terms of "sacrifice". It merely comes with the territory.

An Indian story I read recently in my dear friend Lucy's manuscript: A son was very close to his mother, and she to him. When he finally got married, to a beautiful girl that he loved dearly, the bride grew jealous of the love between mother and son. The bride asked her husband if he would do anything she asked to prove his love for her, his wife. He said yes. "Bring me your mother's liver", she demanded. Reluctantly, he cut out his mother's liver, presumably leaving her lifeless. Walking back home to his wife with the liver, the husband tripped and fell, dropping the liver. At which point the liver gently enquired, "You didn't hurt yourself, did you, son?"

I saw Matthew this afternoon. We had tea together at a local cafe and talked about writing. And spiritual window-shopping. And truth.

## Wednesday 1 December

Phone calls and some levity in the air. In response to some lightweight moaning on my part about having to sleep in the spare room when you're home, you retorted: "I think paying the bills entitles me to the big bed, don't you?"

But later I thought you sounded low and told you so. "I'm alright," you said, "just here in a hotel lobby." The implication? One necessarily sounds low in a hotel lobby?

"Is that woman causing you strife?" I asked. "Want me to get up there and sort her out for you?"

Snorts through the phone. "Irony of ironies", you said.

But I know I won't remain so good-humoured.

## Monday 6 December

And I didn't. Change, change, change. Great sadness this morning during my meditation. Day thirty-nine of my cycle. Still the discomfort in the womb area, the need for a release that doesn't come. Back pains too, though not major. Feeling awash with hormonal activity. Such compassion for you; a strong sense of how you have loved me, still love me. Clear sight of your need to touch, to be close to me, your wanting me and my body's warmth all these years; graphic memories of your loving expression of this. And such sadness at the mystery that seems to drive apart men and women that have borne children together. The mystery of sex.

Is it contempt for male longing? What is it that constitutes the male gaze, the awe they feel at our bodies? and do most women really care? Once we have our children and have reached "a certain age", do we really care if their longing remains intact? Care enough to respond, that is, to meet that need?

If we don't care enough, yet see in men no will to hurt, no spite, but only a driving, driving need for warmth from a woman's body, then we must let them go.

What problems are there, I wonder, that cannot be solved by compassion?

Let him go. And retain his love.

## Tuesday 7 December

I peed myself this morning. For the first time in months. Woke with a full bladder and got up without first battening off all three sphincters. Then in my hurry to the bathroom I let loose a trail of droplets along the hall. Soberly wiped them up, scolding myself, "That's what happens to crones who forget to do their pelvic floor exercises". The drips of wee a sorry testimony to my laxity.

As I sit here writing this I am tightening relaxing tightening relaxing tightening relaxing tightening relaxing tightening...

## Wednesday 8 December

My stomach feels and looks bloated, despite the continued one-day-a-week fast and all the exercise. It's a menstrual bloat. I still feel as though there's a bleed in there wanting to get out. Some cramping discomfort, tiredness, and a return of the type of back pain I've not experienced for some time. But no blood.

In a meditation a few weeks ago I (half-playfully but quite vividly) visualised the last eggs detaching themselves from my ovaries and heading into the sunset. Now I'm wondering ... did I pull it off?

There is also the astrological variable. Feeling rather low and directionless again, I checked to see where transiting Saturn was, knowing it's due to leave the opposition to my Midheaven soon. And lo. It's just gone retrograde, is exact again in a few days, moving off that aspect finally and for the next twenty-eight years just after Christmas. After which, according to Mr Hand and my own corner of the Collective Unconscious, I shall be "on my way up again". Yee-ha.

## Tuesday 14 December

The weekend took us all our separate ways. Me to a seminar about trees. Jack to two days of "cool fun" at James' place. And you to what you yourself called a "boring" Christmas work bash; freely admitted despite the restriction to your honesty imposed by black leather lace-up shoes and sensible tie.

But ah such friends we are, my darling. More and more and more.

To some who do not know us, I have, with just a touch of derring-do, already referred to you as my ex-husband.

Tomorrow I open a separate bank account.

And Jack just asked "Mum, why's there a bed made up in the spare room?"

The reply: "That's where I sleep. I've been sleeping there for a while now".

"What about Dad?"

Without rancour, and with a smile: "He farts and snores and tosses and turns, and the first time I went off to sleep in the spare room I thought it was pretty nice. So I've been in there ever since ... "

He laughed. You can always appeal to Jack's sense of humour. And just as I was going to say, "Dad doesn't mind anyway. We haven't been having sex for a long time. We're more like friends now. It's kind of nice ... " he'd gone off laughing to find you and say, "Poor Dad; Mum's not sleeping with you any more". Then the school bus had to be got and the moment had passed. But it will come again. And Jack and I will talk.

I realise how much less precious I am feeling now about the separation-and-Jack issue. Your honesty with me, your commitment to our son, these have become clear. It is time now. Jack and I will talk.


### Wednesday 15 December

You phoned me from the airport just before boarding your plane to Sydney for the boring (your word) conference. You phoned to ask me whether the phantom period had started yet. It hasn't. Thanks for phoning. You love me, don't you?

## Thursday 16 December

Jack and I alone together at our local restaurant this evening:

**Me:** Do you mind that Dad's away more these days?

**Jack:** Yeah, I sort of do. But then it means I don't have time to get really fed up with him.

**Me:** I know what you mean ... And you know the other day you felt sorry for Dad because I wasn't sleeping with him any more?

**Jack:** Yeah.

**Me:** Well, Dad doesn't mind. We haven't had sex for quite a while now anyway...

**Jack:** Why not?

**Me:** Well, there's no one reason. It's hard to say. People change. And I'm menopausal. For some women, including me, that means they don't much feel like having sex, at least while they're menopausal.

Pause...

**Jack:** But Mum, what if Dad gets another woman?

**Me:** Well ... what are you asking me?

**Jack:** Would you be insulted?

Some quick thinking here—the truth? Yes. Even if Jan leaves you for the other fellow. What else but the truth?

**Me:** Dad already has a girlfriend. I'm not insulted. Dad and I still love one another and are friends.

**Jack:** (Jaw slack with wonder) Who is it?

**Me:** No-one we know. She lives on the Gold Coast.

**Jack:** Has Dad had it off with her?

**Me:** Yes.

**Jack:** I want to meet her! I've got to know who she is in case I bump into her one day and I'm rude to her and she says what's your name and I tell her who I am and SHE'S DAD'S GIRLFRIEND!

**Me:** I don't think she comes down this way much. And if Dad wanted to take you to meet her, I wouldn't mind.

**Jack:** It's so easy for adults!

**Me:** What is?

**Jack:** Finding girlfriends.

**Me:** Do you want one?

**Jack:** Yes.

**Me:** There's no mystery. Just be Jack. Just be honest when you talk to girls. They're human too. Not a different species.

Laughter.

It went so well, so easy. No drama. No apparent fears. Some more easy talk about other things. Then later, feeling heartened and emboldened by his response:

**Me:** One of the reasons we've been talking about sub-dividing the property lately is because Dad has always said he'd like to build a house on that hill to the east—you know? So if he did that he could live up there and you could have two houses to call home.

But his soft rosy face suddenly looked fearful:

**Jack:** No. I don't want that. Why would he do that?

**Me:** (*Band-aiding*) Well ... he's said he might do that ... not for a few years ... it would take time ... so he can have his own space, his own place, but still be with us.

**Jack:** But he wouldn't be with us in a separate house.

**Me:** Separate but close enough for us to walk to and fro. What is it you object to?

**Jack:** We wouldn't be a family then. Families should be together in the same house.

**Me:** There are lots of different ways of being a family. The most important thing that makes a family is loving one another. I don't doubt Dad's love for us, or his promise that he would never separate from us in the way that some dads do.

**Jack:** But I still don't want him to live on the hill. Not while I'm still around.

**Me:** Nothing's going to happen suddenly. And nothing's going to happen without all three of us talking about it.

We meandered into different topics. We were cool. Some laughter. Story-swapping. It was an alright evening after all.

### Friday 17 December

You came home a day early. I was delighted. Jack too. You stepped out of your car, he hugged you immediately and said, friendly-like, "Mum says you've got a girlfriend!" And you said, half-laughing, "Ooh!" And he said he wanted to meet her and you said that might happen and then looked at me and I knew something had changed. "But you're not going to live up on the hill", Jack rattled on, "not while I'm still here." You looked at me again. Yes, we *had* covered a lot of ground in your absence. "If that ever did happen", you said to Jack, "it wouldn't be for ages ... " More hugs and helping you in with your bags, etc.

Later: Jack asleep. We had the fire in the brazier outside — in December! Saturn looking glorious in the west. You said how ironic. Then I knew for sure you'd finished it with Jan — for the moment. Then you said you'd finished it with Jan — for the moment. Why? You said she'd been "screwing around" with her ex. "What d'you mean, screwing around?" I like clarity. You said having sex. I suppose that's clarity. Since when? About a month. Said you'd known, but only now have told her it's you or him. Said you were disappointed in your reaction, not very "skillful" you said, using the Buddhist term: the clinging, the exclusiveness. Meanwhile she's "going through hell", you said, doesn't want to lose you, but can't keep her insistent ex at bay.

We talked about AIDS. Has the guy been sexually active elsewhere? It seems so. You gave her an ultimatum last month: use condoms with him. "I value my life", you told her. She agreed. But you've no way of knowing if they did, you said.

And the ex is there for her. On the spot. Within her reach seven days a week. Not like you, who love us, me and Jack.

Male double standards? I think not. Just life flexing its muscles.

"Maybe I'll find another woman ... " you said. Maybe. But this could always be a problem, couldn't it, my darling, in this era of man-and-woman-as-two-peas-in-a-pod-copulating-at-least-every-day-otherwise-you're-not-getting-enough-and-if-you-don't-want-it-that-much-you-need-therapy-and-while-we're-at-it-let's-get-our-own-home-and-spend-the-rest-of-our-lives-supporting-the-multi-nationals-starting-off-by-getting-that-chocolate-coated-beautifully-wrapped-stereo-system-we-saw-the-other-day-when-we-were-out-and-about-having-a-break-from-the-sex ...

Bitter? No. Not me.

Don't you remember how I hugged you and told you I was genuinely sorry this had happened? I could see your hurt. Feel it.

I love you.

## Saturday 18 December

More talk. Talking therapy. Therapeutic talking. Let's keep it up. Open open open, not close close close. I asked, foolishly for a Buddhist, but perhaps not for a Western Buddhist, "Do you think we'll ever be lovers again?" You said, "It's up to you". Then you said, "I'd be very surprised if we never made love again". A distinction there, between lovers and making love. You grow subtler. I may at times have thought you an oaf, and you thought me a dreamer, but we change, do we not?

## Friday 31 December

Here again among the eucalypts for ten days of meditation and study. Bushfire weather. We drove through blackened bush to get here. The flames crept close to our camp. I saw the sweat, the exhaustion on the firefighters' faces, never before seen at such close quarters. Brave people.

Chittaprabha is here. Coolly inspirational.

## Sunday 9 January 1994

Out now. At a friend's place with Chittaprabha, a timber house surrounded by eucalypts. The fires came close. We are here for moral support. Phone calls to and from you. The first weekend I was away Jan spent with her ex. She's now with you at home, has been there since Wednesday. You say she's close to a nervous breakdown. I wonder, sometimes at our role in all this. You sound quite detached — what you'd hoped to achieve. Said you'd invited her back home after work on Wednesday as you would invite any friend in that amount of trouble with themselves.

## Wednesday 12 January

Reunion with Jack. Such hugs. With you. More hugs. And some gifts for me. But at dinner (out) this evening the father's lack of enjoyment in the son, the father's lack of spontaneity, lack of humour, lack of the spark of life . . . oh dear. I had little to say. You asked, politely I thought, about the retreat. How to share that inspiration with someone who, perhaps, *perhaps* like me, is perhaps, *perhaps* considering that perhaps, *perhaps* it's too late for any rekindling of interest (perhaps).

## Saturday 15 January

Oh dear, oh dear, oh dear. I see I'm still jealous, still clinging, still attached, in spite of all the above fine words. I had sort of thought — and I have to admit this to myself — that you were beginning to "see sense", to see that this person you were involved with led a rather messy and complex life, from which you were now extricating yourself. I had not thought about a return to the status quo (I know in my heart that's not possible), but I had thought that you were thinking of leaving Jan behind and getting on with the simpler life of non-attachment. This thought had been pleasing me these last few weeks.

But now you talk again of a possible long-term relationship and how that could work best if we are all friends, etc., etc. and etc., all sorts of things too tedious to record.

And yet, you say, the relationship's still iffy to the extent that you don't know where you'll be sleeping on Monday night after working up the coast.

Well, you and Jan may be iffy, but your saying this does clarify things for me. I had been happy in your loving phone calls and yes, I had been thinking perhaps we could be in love again in a sort of way. But I'm now feeling distinctly written off, as you talk about your "long-term" relationship.

Wish I could sort out how I really feel about this. God, where does all the accumulated wisdom go at such times? At this point I couldn't even tell you how much I *care* about you disconnecting from my life. Though it could be that tomorrow, or even this after-bloody-noon, I'll have a distinct handle on all of it.

Feeling pre-menstrual. Have missed three periods. Was hoping the ovaries were denuded. Maybe they are ... Anyway ...

George is here. He has brought suitable and timely gifts, as always. How much older he seems to have become, your Dad. In just over a year.

## Thursday 20 January

It is harder with George here. Harder not to be close to you. Not to be our old selves. Remembering how good it was between us. Feeling sorry for myself. Abandoned and Free. Old and On-The-Threshold-Of-My-Life. Do I contradict myself? Very well then ...

We are all away for a week's indulgent holiday come Saturday—you 'n' me, George, Jack and friend Ben.

## Tuesday 25 January

On holiday with you, you who are perfectly within the rights of the evolving-soul not to love me as you have done. You. The father-of-my-son, I thought when I woke up this morning and looked across at you, from my double bed to your double bed, Jack's smooth sprouting ten-year-old arm on the full-blown hairy doormat of your chest.

## Thursday 27 January

Well yes. I suppose we have demonstrated our friendship. On holiday together. You and me. We've been alright in our separate hotel beds. Jack and Ben have run their urgent little bodies through a week of indulgence. George had done what George does best—stayed in step with what's happening and talked about the little things.

When you told me that you had told him about us, just before we left, you know what popped into my sentimental mind? Oh god he's serious — he's actually told his Dad. Ah the chains of conditioned existence! What price all this talk of freedom?

I recall George had looked at me in a particularly kindly way when you returned from your confessional lunch with him, during which you said you had "dated" a couple of other women. (I could have vomited when you used that silly word but I deep-breathed and didn't react. Like the good meditator I have become, I merely observed my own pain and anguish, labelled it PAIN AND ANGUISH, and moved on in full knowledge of my suffering.)

George won't say doodly-squat to me about it. Treads too carefully the well-ploughed field of bourgeois bushido. But I'll talk to him about it before he leaves, support what you've told him about our mutual commitment to his grandson, try to put an old man's mind at rest on that score at least.

I'm wondering if this belly I've grown over the last few months is going to be a permanent fixture.

And I ache, I ache, I ache. Everything from the waist down, traditionally the least conscious part of my body, has been aching. For months. Knees. Toes. Feet. Backs of legs. Fronts of legs. Gurglings and churnings in the abdomen. All this swimming and relaxation on holiday hasn't afforded me the (relatively) pain-free experience of an intensive meditation retreat. But then ... but then ... I haven't had a period in nearly four months.

So.

Maybe.

THIS IS IT!

NO MORE EGGS!

Eggless. Without an ability to create life. How do I feel about this? Fine. I feel fine. In theory. But it could be my biology's in mourning. Is that why I'm so ill-inclined to leap dolphin-like from my bed in the mornings?

And another thing. The urgency around piddling has returned. It subsides if I bend down. In public I am sometimes forced to pretend an itchy ankle or an untied shoelace while I get the pelvic floor up and doing its job again, enabling me thus to walk sedately and with head held high to my goal — the dunny.

Margaret is looking after our animals, our place. I phoned her. "I don't want to go back to the city", she said. I nearly said don't then. Stay with me and we'll be husband-less together. Without domesticity we'll have more time for ourselves and for others. Offer our enormous resources outside the gates of the Nuclear Family. Climb out of our bourgeois ruts and start really giving, loving, nurturing. And playing. Ah yes. Playing. I nearly said that to her.

But only nearly.

## Wednesday 2 February

Wow. The man who never says sorry actually apologised. Trying to talk to you about spending money on maintaining this huge place which it was *your* idea to buy, when I would have been in Elysium with only four hectares ... well, trying to talk to you about spending money proved impossible once again. You adopted that superior lip-curl and asked if it was only the negative aspects of the place I could see.

How did you dare say such a thing when only last night I'd thanked you for a fine holiday, adding, "But for all that, this place is more beautiful, isn't it?" Your power to upset me remains intact. I guess I made that clear, because you actually apologised. You came to see me later as I sat working at my desk. Sorry for upsetting you, you said.

Well, we need to talk about money. I'm meeting half the

costs of the landcare from my meagre earnings, using my cash to keep the triffids from victoriously bursting through our last lines of defence. If you shared my vision we'd have spent—alright I know it's *your* money, but what are you going to do with it? buy an investment unit at a seaside resort?—we'd have spent it on a tractor and together slashed our way through the accursed weeds that ever threaten the saintly, stately trees.

Maybe you only apologised because George is still here and you want to keep me cool. And yes, I'm a cynic. Sometimes.

It's grown harder with George here. There is no warmth or spontaneity between you and your father. You circle one another, perplexed. The only animated conversation is about legacies, about stocks and shares.

You thanked me for being kind to him. What else would I be to an old gentleman with whom there is no true point of contact? Honesty frightens him. Small talk keeps him safe.

What have I done in the past at such times? Times when my cosy self, my everything's-alright-really self has been prodded by life's pitchforks? I've simply got up and moved; like an irritated amoeba I've sought the less gritty part of the pond. My mother was gritty. My childhood was gritty. So I sent out a few pseudopodia to take me away to eminently smoother and duskier unknown lands, where I remained devoid of gritty emotions for some years. The first of many cunning and finely executed moves away from myself. Yes, I've been a good mover.

Then on the very eve of my fiftieth birthday it stuck me in one of those heart-stopping moments of Truth:

I must stay here and not run away from the people I have responsibilities towards, the people capable of making my life uncomfortable. I must stay here and work slowly and quietly and methodically towards fulfilling my myth, which has something to do with helping to nurture the community of human fellow-sufferers by nurturing the land — this land that I find myself taking on more and more responsibility for. I will not abandon it as I sometimes think of doing just so I can say to you, so there arsehole, look what you've made me do now!

## Thursday 3 February

So. You told me this morning you'd spent your nights again with Jan while up the coast. She'd vowed that the ex was truly ex. But whether he was or not would not alter your new-found sense of detachment. You also said for the first time, and quite definitely, that you "couldn't see us being married again ... "

That seems to have shifted something in me. I felt jealousy, admitted jealousy, decided jealousy wasn't doing me any good, decided it was time for me to talk to George too, to reiterate what you'd said: that our marriage as such was over but we were committed to remaining together as friends for the foreseeable future for the sake of our son; that Jack knew about this, knew you had a girlfriend, saw that we still loved one another as friends and did not seem to be threatened by these developments.

George listened quietly, said very little, just that it is the children that suffer most when parents fight, that he was sorry for both of us, that he didn't know who was right and who was wrong — "We're trying not to look at it from the point of view of who's right and who's wrong", I said, and he nodded. Told me some story about a peer of his who said how she couldn't understand "these modern divorces" where the couples are not constantly at one another's throats, as though that were the desirable state of affairs.

That was about it, really.

## *Monday 7 February*

We were doing imprints of our faces during dinner at the Taylors' place when both you and Jack commented on my nose. The wine I'd consumed coloured my judgement of you, not Jack. Only you. We got home late but I was saying my hurt-feelings-piece the moment we were alone. If you had any sensitivity you wouldn't be pointing out my imperfections at such a time blah blah blah ... Didn't know Jack was overhearing. Tears as he put himself to bed.

**Me:** What's wrong?
**Jack:** I'm the one that said you had a big nose first.
**Me:** (*Laughter at self for being fool as well as having big nose.*)
**Jack:** You and Dad are going to break up. If I have to choose which one of you I'm going to live with then I'd rather be dead.
**Me:** (*No more laughter.*) Haven't you seen what friends Dad and I have been to one another lately? Much better friends than in a long time. But what do friends do sometimes? They have differences, they have arguments. Like you and Ben. I started this one because I'm feeling over-sensitive after drinking too much wine. Booze does that sort of thing. What I said to Dad was daft and I'll apologise to him for it. I won't say there won't be other times when Dad and I have skirmishes but just remember, we're not at war, we're just human. We make mistakes, say silly things. Even the wisest old people sometimes say silly things.

And there is no way Dad and I would make you choose between us. That's cruel, it's like using your child as a weapon. We both love you, and that means your happiness is as important to us as our own.

He listened. Nodded occasionally. I finished: "We'll talk with Dad about it tomorrow, eh?" Another nod. Then him: "We have to talk about getting a tractor too ... " Then sleep ... child-sleep.

And you were good, what you said to him, the following evening, last night, about as far as conventional marriage was concerned you and I had already broken up. "But look at us, Jack, here together, working together happily all day on the land, going to the beach with you and Grandpa ... "

Then the girlfriend. He needed to know about the girlfriend. Would Dad get to love her so much that he would leave us in the end? You told him again that he was Number One, his happiness; you had no intention of leaving either of us.

Alright. Time for me to interject: You know, Jack, I don't want to think of Jan as the enemy of our family. If she and Dad want, she could be part of our family. We could be friends with her.

**You:** Would you like to meet her sometime, Jack?

**Jack:** Yes. (*Then thoughtful.*) But I think I should meet her first, at her place, rather than have her come here. Then after I've met her she could come here and meet Mum.

You commented later, and I think you're right, that you thought Jack said that because he was beginning to see himself in a different light, as the — was "cement" the word you used? — the cement of the family. Well now. How often have I said that sex is not necessarily the only force that might bind a family together? A sensitive ten-year-old might do just as well.

## Sunday 13 February

Serious pelvic-floor exercises. Unruly thinking swinging from "Oh I do feel sorry for that poor woman Jan, lumbered with your ego", to "Thank you, my darling, for all the kindness over the years". Essential not to respond to such jumble. Just keep returning to the still point.

### Thursday 17 February

Arid mornings. Waking to no man. No big-heaving-body-warmth. No reliable, insistent arms pulling me into a cuddle. I lie alone. And I think, I am celibate. Dessicated. A celibate, dessicated old lady with green still somewhere in her twigs.

### Friday 18 February

You talk now of studying hypnotherapy, having consulted a hypnotherapist some time ago when things were bad for you, and found it helpful. This is a big change for you, removed from the mainstream, from the financial markets. You talk of lack of interest in your work, of your inability to kowtow to an authority you now describe as "contemptible". Our friendship deepens. Becomes more real.

### Thursday 24 February

I was just thinking about my response to the news of Steve and Heather breaking up. I said, "And not so long ago he was telling us how much in love with her he was ... " And your response? You said, "Perhaps he is. Perhaps he is ... "

### Monday 28 February

I get up, do yoga, meditate. Easy-easy when you sleep alone. And I make my bed tidily, straight away, before the yoga. I notice you are making your bed too, no longer leave it for me not to do. How ... liberating.

## Tuesday 1 March

You say you haven't "progressed as much" as me. That you may well still be jealous if I find myself a man. Progress? What's that? It's not linear, that's for sure. I know because when you phoned today to suggest Jack stayed with friends this weekend so you could invite Jan here while I was off on my weekend meditation retreat, I thought, "What cheek! What nerve!" Then I said why not leave it till the weekend I'm in Sydney, since Jack didn't see you all last week. I said that calmly, while feeling ... what? Jealous, though I turned it into concern for Jack, which was not entirely fabricated. Was half the truth.

I know you listen to my concerns for Jack and I appreciate it. But where's the dividing line between motherly concern and jealousy? In the midnight of my thinking — your phone call — that line became suddenly clear.

## Thursday 3 March

You're still overnighting at Louise's when you're away up the coast, still sorting out your relationship with Jan. This sorting out, which includes not sleeping at her place, has been going on some time. I asked you, "How are you managing without sex?" You said, "Oh we had sex last week. It was great. We seem to be sexually compatible".
Oh.

## Saturday 12 March

**You:** What's the difference between telling people we're separated and telling them we're unmarried?

**Me:** We're not separated. We still function as a family, economically, to an extent socially, and as far as Jack's relationship to us both is concerned, emotionally. The words we use are important. I don't want to think of us as separated because Jack needs us both, as family, as a unit. We have to stay a family until he no longer needs that.

**You:** I see. I understand.

So do I, now. And thanks for asking. I didn't know the answer myself till I heard the question.

## Friday 25 March

Resting with the alone-ness of no sex, no man in bed. Sitting on my own knee. Crying on my own shoulder, observing my solitude. Without meditation it would be hard. Without friends even worse. And without work it would be impossible. My students! Hugs at the recent conclusion of a course. And written messages of love. They say I am marvellous. Yet like them I struggle. I struggle so much, in my mind. They do not know the bamboo-spiked pits my mind falls into when left alone without Awareness to keep the way clear.

## Tuesday 5 April

A visit to the menopause clinic in town and a conversation with the female doctor:

**Me:** I consider I'm doing alright compared with others I know. I exercise a lot, swimming, living on a farm. I'm mindful of diet, don't smoke, drink only very moderately. But still I'm not the woman I was. I was wondering if the discomfort to the point of pain in the abdomen, which has been going on for some time, the aching joints—especially knees and especially in the morning, the odd sort-of vaginal infection, and the increased PMT could be easily dealt with? I went to the forum you people organised last year and know something about the options.

She asked me a lot of questions and slapped my wrists for the years of forgetting pap smears (hate the term, sounds dirty) and mammograms (hate that too, sounds monumental), did the smear, examined my breasts, wrote the referral for the x-ray, said everything seemed fine and then:

**Doctor:** You'll have come to your own conclusions at the forum, so you can take away what I'm going to suggest to you and think it through as you will. Even though you're feeling well compared with other women your age, you clearly want to feel better, so you may like to consider therapy for a while, and see how you go with it.

**Me:** (*Marginally aghast*) You mean HRT?

**Doctor:** Yes.

**Me:** I didn't think my symptoms were severe enough to merit an intervention like that.

**Doctor:** It's a personal choice. A lot of women without severe symptoms take it simply to feel better.

**Me:** And do they?

**Doctor:** Generally speaking, yes.

**Me:** (*Silence.*)

**Doctor:** Think about it. You can try it for a few months and see if it helps. You don't have to stay on it if you decide not to. Think about it and come back to see me in six weeks' time. We'll have your various test results by then. In the meantime you might like to try this (*holds up thin plastic tube with little plunger at one end and little white tablet at the other*). It's an oestrogen pessary. You insert the oestrogen tablet into the vagina, one a day for a week or so, then one every two days. It helps oestrogenise the vagina and may ease the vaginal and other discomfort you've been experiencing.

**Me:** Alright (*taking script and leaving*).

## Saturday 9 April

Our Jack had his eleventh birthday with his friend, Andrew in Sydney. The first birthday away from home. And Pauline was here, she who helped me breathe through Jack's heaving into the world, into drought-ridden Victoria all those years ago ... crossed the planet, she did, my little nurse, my oldest friend, came from England to give me a hug on my fiftieth, bringing the laconic and absurdly English Ollie, and their two young children. And it was you that helped engineer the surprise, with such love and care and patience. Such quietness. Even Jack picked up enough not to spill the beans. You may never know what that meant to me.

But ah that old Buddha ... he's a wily one.

You went away to Jan's for Easter, the relationship being officially on again. With Jack away too, I was to have space to write. But there was none. The word processor synchronistically went bung and left me with Pauline and Memories.

And left you with recent relevations:

**Me:** (*On the phone, when you were due home last Wednesday, not having seen you for a week*) I'm not interested in how you are. I've lost that feeling of friendship. I'm feeling all pent up, angry. Just thought you might like to know, it'll explain why you won't get much of a welcome this evening. Kathy's asked me out for an Indian meal, so I'll only be here for a little while after you get home. You might want to organise dinner elsewhere.

**You:** You're feeling anger at me?

**Me:** Yes.

**You:** That's understandable.

**Me:** Is it?

**You:** Yes. I've been thinking about you a lot. Concerned about you. I thought it would be harder for you with Pauline here.

**Me:** Well it is.

And then later, on Thursday, I spent half the day lying around crying. Felt it incumbent upon me that evening, after we had enjoyed a pleasant meal (cooked by me) during which I'd felt suitably distanced from reacting to my anger, to tell you that I couldn't help feeling you were a fool.

You didn't deny it.

**You:** I've been doing a lot of thinking lately, about my relationship to you, to Jack, to Jan.

I didn't probe. And you didn't volunteer. I managed to bite back the words of the Chinese saying:

*If you don't change direction you are going to wind up where you are going.*

You start your hypnotherapy course today. Now there's a change.

## Sunday 10 April

The tears of last week were not entirely nostalgic, but also partially hormonal, it seems. A smear of blood on the nightie this morning, five months after my vision of denuded ovaries.

I wondered if those natty-looking little oestrogen pessaries were responsible, but I'd only inserted the first one last night, and last week's tears are evidence of hormonal movement way before the pessary fact.

So there you are. A textbook example of the drop in oestrogen production. Five months without a bleed, thinking "welcome to the cash savings on tampons and pads", then here-we-are-again.

## Wednesday 13 April

It lasted only the usual two days, a little heavier than it used to be, though not "heavy".

## Wednesday 20 April

Twists and bumps in my life but I stay mostly upright, listing only occasionally and then discreetly. I say, yes of course this is happening now but it will change and as far as I'm concerned such thoughts indicate a kind of progress. When you phoned this morning it was to see if I was still coping with the English influx. You mentioned you'd made a bid on a house up the coast, an investment property you called it, a plan you've been formulating for some time. You'll let it to Jan "at the market price". How convenient, I thought, when you first told me you were thinking of it. How convenient, I thought this morning, too. Sometimes I think I loathe you for not sharing my vision of making something special of this land we have here. For not working with me on it, for not helping me plant a little seed in our son that will reveal the beauty and the necessity of loving the land.

## Wednesday 27 April

So you bought your house *so* conveniently close to where Jan lives and now you will be her landlord too. At this moment, and I recognise that this moment will pass, but nonetheless at this moment I have to say it: I hate you.

**Me:** I feel outraged at what you've done. Even though you told me you were thinking about it ages ago and I didn't respond much one way or another, just felt it was your business I suppose. But now it's done I feel betrayed and used and abandoned and I'm thinking, "He's bought her a house with the money from the house in Sydney that I—ME ME ME—that I made into a beautiful home, helped to make saleable etc., etc., blah, blah ... "

A pained look on your face. An effort of mind to snatch at possibilities of logic in my thinking. But sometimes there *is* no logic in my thinking. Ever since this started last Easter, my thinking has been a battleground, strewn on the one hand with the corpses of my Conditioning, such as:

I Must Have A Rhett Butler
and
My Marriage Is My Security;

invaded on the other by thoughts bent on reviving that conditioning—thoughts like:

Why Should I Make It Easy For Him?
Who Does He Think He Is?
He Can't Do This To Me!
and
You Fucking Bastard!

You kept silence. And I ... what did I do? ... I shrugged my shoulders.

## Thursday 28 April

The day passed in a flurry of work and a kind of success, and just as I was enjoying the lovely dinner cooked by your hand, Jack said, "Guess what, Mum?"

**Me:** Tell me.
**Jack:** I'm meeting Dad's girlfriend next weekend.
**Me:** (*Looking at you*) Oh.

**Jack:** It's the (*something-or-other*) soccer match.
**Me:**(*Looking at you*) I would have appreciated being told before this.
**You:** I'm sorry, I was planning to tell you. Jack and I were going to the match from way back and I got four tickets for whoever else may have wanted to go. I didn't know till the other day that Jan and her son had decided to go. Then Jack asked me if he was going to meet her that day and I told him yes. I was going to tell you yesterday, but I didn't think you'd want to hear it because you were in such a bad space.
**Me:** I'm in a worse one now.
**Jack:** Don't argue.
**Us:** We're not.
**Me:** (*Mopping up*) I appreciate being told when you or Dad or both of you are going to be away. I have outside interests too, and maybe would like to make arrangements to see friends that day, you know ...

Jack went off to watch the wondrous David Attenborough telling about the even more wondrous emperor penguins of Antarctica and I moved into a quietly controlled how-dare-you mode. You could have told Jack that Jan hadn't decided yet, only a little white lie to save both of us the angst. You fool. You've no idea about people. You kept saying sorry.

## Friday 29 April

And then this morning, after my meditation, I was thinking I never wish to part company with you, to see you drive away, on bad terms. Because people die, you know. They die all the time, any time. And you could drive away with my anger and hatred on your tail and die. And what then could I say to you to make up for it, my friend?

Because this much I do know, that we can live with people and live with people and still they elude us. It may be that all I will ever really know about you is that you were a good provider to me and my baby. And I thank you for that.

So I was approaching you to give you a silent hug when Jack came behind me and put his arms around us both, saying, "I bond you both together", and the three-way hugs were real and long lasting. You said something, can't remember it, something nice. I told Jack not to take it all on himself.

**Jack:** But I worry.
**Me:** About what?
**Jack:** That you'll split up.
**You:** What does that mean to you? Splitting up?
**Jack:** That one of you will go away.
**You:** Look Jack, as far as conventional marriage is concerned, Mum and I have already "split up". But look at us. We're both still here, still friends, still a family.
**Me:** It doesn't work well all the time, Jack. Like last night. I was angry at Dad. Sometimes it's really hard. Sometimes it's great. Mostly it works fine.

He nodded, was happy with that.

Stop press: a sudden call from Leanne to tell me that she observed her dog some time ago panting to cool itself down, tried it on her next hot flush and lo! it worked. That was months ago. Since then it's not failed for her or her friends. "It can be just a discreet pant behind the hand if you want, but it works! You cool down!"

Perhaps not so surprising when you consider the use of breath in childbirth, the mind paying attention to the breath, not the pain. Here the mind pays attention to the breath, not the heat.

If ever I get a hot flush, I'll try it.

## Sunday 8 May

Two weeks of feeling my period is about to start. Two weeks on a merry-go-round of dislike for you, compassion for you, dislike for you ... Last night's conversation, following a day of soccer and horseriding for you and Jack and Jack's young friends, and a day of killing weeds for me:

**Me:** You've seemed rather unhappy these last few weeks. It's not just your sore bones either.

**You:** Bad week at work, study. Not living up to my expectations of myself. When I was a kid I always dreaded mediocrity. But I think that's what I've become. Mediocre.

**Me:** An awful thing to think about yourself.

**You:** Well.

**Me:** A while ago you said you'd be surprised if we never made love again. Do you still think that?

**You:** Less and less.

**Me:** Same here. Will we stay friends?

**You:** I think so. I hope so. If I can support you in making this place into what you envision, something for the community, something beautiful for people, plants and animals, then that'll be my contribution to the planet.

We had a cuddle in your bed this morning, the first in a long time. I figured you needed a friend. I crawled in and warmed myself on you and told you (again) about the Saturn cycle in your chart, how the time is right for looking inward, reviewing your life, and having to slow down to do this. How the same transit affected me over the last three or so years. How it needs to be acknowledged. How you need to simplify your life in order to really look within. Your decision to study hynotherapy at this time in your life is not *merely* coincidental; it is *meaningfully* coincidental.

I told you I thought what you were trying to do in keeping your family together was far from mediocre. Where many men would walk away from a marriage they no longer felt happy with, you have taken a more creative, and perhaps more difficult path.

You said thanks for the friendship. Hugged me hard.

Well there it is. As well as hating you, my friend, I love you.

It's Mother's Day today! And how fortunate that these commercial pressures mean nothing to me because today Jack meets Jan. At a soccer match. While I stay home, plan lessons, and write, write, write.

## Monday 9 May

Jack said she reminded him of my friend Margaret. Well, could be a lot worse.

## Saturday 14 May

Following a week of PMT and of mostly hating you, the bleed finally started, a decision was finally made. When I see the doctor at the menopause clinic this coming Wednesday I'll tell her to start me on a course of hormone replacement therapy. And then. We'll see.

## Wednesday 18 May

This evening I took a little blue tablet before going to bed. There are more blue tablets in the packet, followed by some white ones, followed by some red ones. By the time I get to the red ones, I should have a "light" bleed. Once a month.

It's a very moderate dosage. The doctor said she didn't envisage me being on HRT "for decades", that perhaps a year or so of therapy would help me through the symptoms of lowered energy, PMT and aches and pains I have been experiencing. Made another appointment with her, to report in a month from now, and went off holding my little plastic wheel of red-white-and-blue tabs in my trusting hand.

I wonder if they'll reawaken my snoozing libido? And what if they do? Will it be you, Noel, I jump upon, or will it be somebody else? Look in two months from now.

## Sunday 29 May

Woke this morning with less stiffness in joints. Is it HRT or my new futon?

Busy busy. Landcare. Questioning my own teaching methods. Am I doing my creative best for my students, or am I stuck in thirty-year-old methodology?

Trying to cut down, to slash to 200 manuscript pages, this rambling behemoth of a journal because I think it might interest others, might be publishable. What do you think, Noel? Would you mind? I ought to show it to you first. Are you ready to look back in this way, over the last year-and-a-half?

## Wednesday 15 June

Looking back over this journal. Trying to pull together an Introduction to it. Trying to follow each of the threads that have tangled through my life, so I can identify just one that tells me why I married you. Forlorn enterprise! Impossible! Even if I find one that seems to be leading my groping self somewhere, I know that by tomorrow morning it will have frayed away to nothing.

I recall that when we were first together I said I could live happily in a shack with you and we could do Good Works. How free I felt. Not like now. Not like these last few weeks.

Now I wake up in a cage of mainstream comfort. The

person rattling my bars is you—and you're on the outside, in your own cage admittedly, reaching through, jiggling me up and down and saying, "Well, then, get on with it! You wanted to serve the community instead of exploiting it—go for it!"

But I didn't expect to miss you this much, didn't expect to miss being the nuclear family we had become, with all its comfort, its privacy, its ease. You asked if it would be OK if Jack overnighted with you occasionally at Jan's when there was a sporting event he might like to go to up the coast. In response, I asked you to give me more time to get used to the idea. I saw it as a further step in the expropriation of my son rather than a further step along the path to greater freedom for us all. I saw Jack enjoying the life of trashy video-parlour temptations and fast food, and being bored here alone with me, or outraged with me if I were to share this space with homeless teenagers and/or peace-loving meditators. Though the doors have always been open to his friends, he has not grown up in a truly sharing household. Will I drive my boy away with my visions of community?

I am in a cleft-stick. Faced with a choice that may lead me into very different concepts of family, by way of sharing much more of myself with the wider community.

The HRT. The HRT. I've now been on it for a month. Slight, very slight, breast tenderness for the first few weeks. Gone now. Still some PMT, to the point where all my good plans fell to the bottom of the pit of my alone-ness and it was an effort to be civil to you. That passed too. But then, when I was half way through the red tablets with the very low oestrogen (at mid-bleed), came that venomous headache on Sunday afternoon. I lay outside on the banana chair for four hours, drinking in the clean air and the crystal sounds and lo, the pain drained away. Then we went to the movies.

The doctor at the menopause clinic said the headache could have been brought on by the lowered oestrogen at the end of the sequence of tablets, and did I want a slightly higher dosage at that point for next month? We can tailor the dosage to individual needs, she said. No, I'll continue this way for the coming month. If I get headaches again at the end, we'll change it then.

**Doctor:** Any other differences you've noticed?

**Me:** It's marginal, but my joints don't feel quite so stiff in the mornings when I get out of bed. Energy level about the same. Certainly not lower.

**Doctor:** Well, that can be significant. Some women do have lowered energy at first, before they start to experience the benefits.

Another recent conversation, this time with you:

**You:** (*Handing me the Bankcard invoice*) Which of these is yours?

**Me:** We haven't really broken it up that way in the past—you always paid the Bankcard bills. And I was never exactly profligate with the plastic. Remember?

**You:** Well now that you're generating income I think you should pay for your items.

**Me:** But what's changed? I've always generated income.

**You:** Not for the last few years.

**Me:** I didn't earn as much when we first moved up here as in Sydney. You know the reasons. But that's changing now and I'm getting more and more teaching work. Let's be honest about this: the reason you're putting this out now is because I'm not having sex with you any more. I'm no longer your sexual partner; you've found another one. So your attitude towards paying for certain things on my behalf has changed. Isn't that right?

**You:** You should pay for the things you buy for work purposes, like petrol. You can claim on that.

**Me:** (*Checking down the list*) What else?

**You:** This book. What's that?

**Me:** A teaching book.

**You:** You should pay for that and claim on it.

**Me:** What else do you want me to pay for? The only other thing that's mine on this list is the optometrist's bill, for my reading glasses. Shall I pay for that?

**You:** You tell me what you think's fair.

**Me:** Well, it hasn't been an issue before. I'm not sure. But I'll pay the optometrist. And what about my dentist? I'll be seeing him soon.

**You:** Yes, if you want to pay him, that's fine.

**Me:** But will you pay Jack's dentist's bill?

**You:** Yes.

**Me:** OK. Anything else you want to discuss about money?

**You:** No.

It was quite amiable. But it left me with images of sex and money vying for space in my mind that night.

### Monday 20 June

Yesterday morning, early, you were sitting looking into the fire that you'd lit in the living room. I handed you this journal, with its introduction. It didn't take you long to read. Just two sittings. When you finished it you thanked me for keeping the record. No, there was nothing in it that offended you. "And you write well", you said. We hugged.

### Sunday 10 July

Don't know about this low oestrogen dosage I'm on. Doesn't seem to have made a difference to the customary one day of PMT. I really let it rip last weekend. You sulked at me on Saturday night for using your home-made mitre box as fuel for the fire. Honestly, it just looked like a couple of bits of wood nailed together. You didn't need to sulk at me. I don't expect you to give me a bad time about *anything* these days, because I'm trying so hard not to give you the bad time I sometimes (quite possibly mistakenly) think you deserve.

I could see the grey cloud descend over your head as you lowered yourself into your newspaper, mocked by the flames dancing around your mitre box. I felt the needle points of anger shooting from you. They whizzed through me and suddenly I was banging around the washing up, I became a-machine-for-banging-around-the-washing-up-and-slamming-drawers-shut. There was nothing in my life but this. No other point to make. No room for compromise. Definitely no prisoners. "What's the matter with you?" you asked, ingenuously.

**Me:** You wanna know! You really wanna know!
**You:** Yes!
**Me:** Well, it's this. How dare you be angry with me! I didn't know it was your bloody mitre box! You've no right to be angry with me! I don't bloody deserve it!

You accepted my anger. You argued. You shouldn't have done that. When you don't accept something from a person, it still belongs to them.

Jack cried. I went to him. He pulled us together. We said sorry. God. What progress have I made? It was a PMT outburst that virtually opened this journal nearly two years ago.

Given the fragility of my family situation and the sensibilities of my son, a case exists for upping my dosage of distilled horse's urine. It may keep me from growing extended canines and hair on my back once a month.

The following day:

**Me:** The way I carried on last night wasn't characteristic was it?
**You:** No, it wasn't.

**Me:** If it ever happens again, I'd like you to do something for me.

**You:** What?

**Me:** I'd like you to put your arms around me even as I'm yelling and ask me when my period's due ... I had menstrual cramps this morning.

**You:** Hasn't the HRT had the desired effect?

**Me:** Nope. Not on that score. Also, I had a headache during the last period. Two good reasons for asking the doctor for a higher dosage.

Which I did, a few days later. Combined continuous HRT is what I'll pop into myself on my fourth month of experimentation, which means: no bleeds, and thus no PMT, and you don't risk being accused of patronising me by complying with my request and asking if my period's due next time I yell, *You really wanna know what's wrong!*

Maybe I wouldn't consider continuous therapy if I hadn't had that six-month hiatus in the bleeds. Inside this HRT-driven-bleeder is a woman bereft of eggs, bereft of the need-to-bleed.

Maybe.

Anyway.

I start it in a few weeks.

Looking back at this journal also reminded me of my one-day-a-week fasts. They went by the proverbial board. Though I'm still juicing carrots, celery, fruits, and eating raw more than I otherwise might do.

The supplements, even the evening primrose, I now take only sporadically. But in general I feel physically much better than I've felt in three years. The healing in the back continues. I am much more physically active. Lots to do on the land. Still the odd swim. Can teach all day without needing to fling myself down on the bed when I get home.

It's not just the HRT. This process began before that.

## Thursday 21 July

Some time has passed. And I see your study of hypnotherapy quietening you, making you more reflective. "Interesting", you've been saying of your experimental visits to a local hypnotherapist. "Interesting to see how she does things, with me on the client-end."

But not tonight. You didn't say "interesting" tonight. Tonight you cried. Told me she had done age-regression with you. Taken you back to when you were two years old. You had always roused my curiosity by not being able to remember anything of your childhood until about the age of ten. I had suspected it. Suspected the happy laughing North American Dream Family in the eight-millimetre film shows. Those were the images you used to supplant your fear.

You spoke to me about the terror you had experienced while under hypnosis. A memory of being two years old and left alone among strangers for two weeks in a hospital, strangers who were preparing you to have your arm amputated. *Eosinophilic granuloma* it was. Your Mum didn't come for the whole two weeks. "Why not?" you asked your Dad on the phone, after the hypnotherapy session. Because, he said, she had the two other children to care for. And your Dad didn't come. "Why not?" The doctors had advised against it, he told you. The visits would have been too upsetting for all concerned.

So your parents obeyed while you sobbed your heart into withdrawal from them and your home. So much so that after the reprieve came and you were sent home with both arms intact, you did not know them, did not want to know them.

And, you told me, sobbing again forty-one years later, you see now and for the first time what this has made of your life. In your fear of being abandoned again by loved ones, you have sought out friends, men and women, that you felt could be made dependent upon you. Dependent upon your strength. Your capability. Your ability to attract money.

"My best friends and the few serious girlfriends have all been poor", you said. "No money. They have been the only people I've been attracted to. And I've made them depend on me."

With your kindness you've bound people to you. Did it to me, you said. Talked about how terrified you were of losing me. Then, as you saw me growing in individuality and independence, saw I no longer needed you, you pushed me away.

"And now what am I doing?" you asked me. "The same thing with Jan. The same responses I had when I fell in love with you. I was terrified you would go back eventually to your ex-boyfriend in London. Terrified when you wrote to him from New Guinea, received letters from him. Though I never said a word. And now, with Jan. When her ex-husband phones, and when she sometimes has lunch with him, I'm terrified again ..."

You cried and cried. "I'm sorry", you kept saying. "I made you dependent on me and then I rejected you. I did to you what was done to me ..."

And I? I have known the truth of your kindly engineering. But to hear you speak it tonight is astounding. You have cared so little for the life of inner reference, mistrusted it, mistrusted it in me, who has pursued it quietly and without drama. Yet here tonight it turns its mirror upon you and you are distraught at the image you see.

And I feel now doubly bereft.

Your truth surrounds me now with ... nothing.

Your truth is a vacuum.

I am left without the doubts, the compromises, the half-measures and the denials that accompanied me down the years. I am left without the questions that curtailed my Dreaming: "What if he knows best?" "See how strong and capable he is, see how dependable ... what if? ... what if he's right?"

And into my vacuum your voice came again: "You always told me I was a worrier, too anxious, too hungry. You saw that when I didn't. And I've messed up your life ..."

But I said "no" to that. I can't think in that way. "I made my choices", I said. "You *were* my life. You still are. How could it be otherwise? There's no blame. I don't feel like blaming ..."

After all, what is it, this blaming, blaming, blaming our litigious society encourages us to fall into?

As if life held no mystery.

As if life were a court case.

## Sunday 31 July

"I want to fix it", you had also said of your benign manipulation of loved ones.

"Fix it—meaning what?" I asked.

"Fix it. Deal with it. Stop doing it. Through hypnotherapy."

"That could take time", I offered.

"Hypnotherapy's fast", you told me. "It's known to be one of the fastest of the therapies." And here I thought, trust Noel to choose "the fastest of the therapies". What happened to your slow-and-steady meditation practice, you oaf?

Jack spent last weekend with you at Jan's. There was a basketball match. When you returned Sunday evening he smiled. Held me tight. Said he had a nice time. At dinner you mentioned you would be up the coast again this coming weekend, for a big bank do on Saturday the thirtieth.

**Jack:** But you'll be back Saturday night?
**You:** No. It's not worth all the driving. I'll stay at Jan's till Wednesday.

I felt something go through Jack. I looked at you. You didn't notice. I busied myself with something, came back into the room, Jack had left his dinner, was sitting on your lap, arms tight round your neck, tears. "The weekends are the best time ..." he was saying. You were backtracking, wondering what you'd said, seeing "what could be done ..."

He insisted on your staying with him when he went to bed; fell asleep in your cuddles.

You left him. "Didn't know it would have that effect", you told me.

**Me:** Your timing could be better.
**You:** What do you mean?
**Me:** Don't you think it's been a strain for him, being with you at Jan's this weekend? Despite the brave face he puts on. No matter how nice Jan is, or nice she is to him, what he wants more than anything at the moment is for us two to be together again as his family. And here we are, being a family again over the dinner table, and it looks like you can't wait to tell us next weekend's off.

## Monday 1 August

You phoned today to tell me what the doctor said about your sore throat and your tendency to have choking bouts.

You treat me just like a friend.

Brave faces have prevailed. Except on Sunday when I picked up Jack from James's place after my weekend of writing and his of play and yours of the Gold Coast, I guess I let the face drop.

**Jack:** Is something wrong, Mum?
**Me:** Why do you ask?
**Jack:** The way you look.
**Me:** I'm feeling a bit sad.

**Jack:** What about?

**Me:** About us. About Dad.

**Jack:** Yeah. Me too.

**Me:** How was it for you, last weekend at Jan's?

**Jack:** It was kind of weird.

**Me:** How?

**Jack:** Because it was Dad and Jan, and not Dad and you.

**Me:** Was she nice to you?

**Jack:** Yes.

**Me:** Could you get to like her?

**Jack:** Well it might be a bit hard, because I sort of think that she took Dad away from you. But that's not really true is it?

**Me:** Not exactly. It's not that simple.

**Jack:** It was weird last weekend because it was the first time. I suppose after a while I'd get used to it though.

**Me:** Yes. I think we're both still struggling with it, you and I. Sometimes I still cry, still can't quite believe it.

**Jack:** I hoped at first that Dad would leave her and be with us again all the time. But I don't think that'll happen now.

**Me:** Neither do I. And even if they did break up, I don't think I could return to our old married relationship anyway. In some ways I feel like I'm coming out of a tight, hard chrysalis. And that's going to be better for us all ... maybe.

**Jack:** And the sooner we start accepting it and just getting on with it ... I sort of say to myself now ... well that's the way it is. Can't fight it. No point in fighting it. We'll all be unhappy then. Let's just make the best of it ...

Babes and sucklings ...
Babes and sucklings ...

Interesting, some friends' reactions to the news of your revelations under hypnosis. One friend said that hypnotherapy is known for plunging people into the deep end of their sub-conscious before they are ready, because such traumatic memories should only be uncovered gradually.

And she said, "If he wants to talk about it, I'm here ..."

Another, and quite different reaction, was: "Well, it took your growth as a woman, a fifty-year-old woman, to get him to question his marriage, turn his back on it, and take his own road. He's begun it now. He's on his path. He's started his gig. Thanks to you."

Yet another was, "Whichever way you look at it, he wants to have his cake and eat it."

## Friday 5 August

A dream last night. I am in a cafe/bar with Jack. He's got his machete. He keeps whirling it above his head, playing at warriors. I keep telling him to put it politely upon the table. He gets difficult about it. I suddenly feel tired of trying to be mother and father to a soon-to-be-pubescent hero. I tell him if he continues being macho I'll have to withdraw from motherhood, let him go his own way, because I can't teach him about being a male. He gets up and goes downstairs to the bar. I tell the waiter, "There's a boy downstairs, eleven years old, I just left him, I can't be his mother any more, he can do what he likes. I've had enough. His name's Jack ..." The waiter looks aghast.

I go downstairs, have decided to leave. I just see Jack on one of the benches. A lot of other boys, some bigger than him, are sitting around him, and he is sort of buried beneath them. He's laughing and talking. They're all drinking, and I see with distress a bottle of booze in front of Jack, which he reaches for. I can't stop myself from going over to him and saying, "I'm leaving now ...", half-expecting him to come with me. But he doesn't. I hang around. Then I realise good friends live nearby. I say to Jack, "I might phone Sal and ask her to come and check later that you're alright. You could even sleep at their place." He just shrugs.

Then one of the older boys starts mocking me. I realise

my jumper is pulled right up and my breasts exposed. "Look at those tits!" the older boy giggles. I pull down my jumper and give the kid a good shove. I barely make an impression. He feels rock hard. "What a hard little thing it is!" I say foolishly, and a lot of the boys start laughing and making sexual allusions to "hard things".

I sweep from the place in impotent rage and hear Jack say, "Don't you be mean to my Mum. She's really nice ..."

Outside the cafe/bar I collapse in absolute sorrow, feeling the presence of all these desperate and parentless boy-children around me, plucking at me, appealing dumbly for help. And I sob over and over to you, Noel, who in the dream I see as having left your son and therefore *all* sons: "Why did you do this? Why did you do this?"

I wake crying.

I think of the street kids I've been meeting these last few months. Their stories differ; their suffering has sprung from a variety of dark places. But there is one arena they are all familiar with, the failure of their parents. Fighting parents. Alcoholic parents. Abusive parents. No parents. One overloaded parent. Parents that for whatever reason can't cope.

These insane-looking kids, their features pierced by metal, they are our fruit and we have failed them. Yet still they survive. There is a light inside them, and their strength is remarkable.

### Saturday 13 August

You are holidaying and watching basketball in Canberra next week with Jan and her son. You invited Jack and he has accepted ("If it's alright with Mum ...").

Yes. It's alright with Mum. Dad has two homes now. Two families. We may yet become a blend.

Noel, I'm starting to lose sight of my address to you in

this journal. There was a kind of ending in your actually reading the thing. Now it's becoming a discourse with myself. Time to cease and desist. Stand and deliver. Send it away to be read by editors. There's not one nasty thing they might say about it that I haven't already thought of. One being, "What's the point?"

Hard to answer that. There have been lots of points over the past two years.

Pick your own.

I want to be writing about other things. I want to continue the children's novel. And to write community things. I want to use some of this twentieth-century technology that has brought us information-overload, the technology that has brought us "brain fade" and helped turn people from being interested in one another. We can use that same behemoth to network our local-ness. And I am becoming supremely local.

And some of my mythic things may yet be done. I'm not running with Hollywood and calling this a happy ending. Don't get me wrong, Noel. Stories don't end. The Buddha himself said something about each moment being the result of every other moment since the beginning of time.

Stories never end. Even if journals have to.

# Not a Conclusion

When you write, you lay out a line of words. The line of words is a miner's pick ... You wield it, and it digs a path you follow. Is it a dead end, or have you located the real subject? You will know tomorrow, or this time next year.

Annie Dillard
*The Writing Life*

## January 1995

Jan's eyes are brown. Soft brown and lit from behind. They remind me of the Indian story about God getting fed up with whingeing humanity and confiding to the Devil that He was thinking of taking Himself off to the nether reaches of the universe. "Even out there they'll still find you, eventually", says the Devil knowingly. There is a pause. God nods. "Tell you what", says the wily fallen angel, "why don't you just hide yourself behind their eyes? They'll never think of looking for you there."

The light of kindness was the first thing I saw, meeting her as I did outside the renovated barn, where Noel has now taken up part-time residence. "There's Jan, Mum, there's Jan, there's Jan", breathed Jack, nudging me from my car, wary, and bound steadfast to his own seat. What, I wondered, does he expect me to do?

Relief was what I felt. A falling away of all imaginings. Facing a fellow human being who smiled and said quietly, "Hello". Not a Hollywood bimbo. Not "beautiful" in the silly sense. Not the "other" woman. But a fellow traveller, touching gently upon the complicated things of life.

And I saw then, more clearly than at any other time in my adulthood, even when I was in the throes of writing this journal, that my real values have always been aesthetic, not pragmatic. Pragmatism works well for some of us, but is less necessary for others. I marvel when I meet young adults who seem to know truly how to be themselves, who have held fast to the child in their hearts.

The realisation that my pragmatism had finally come to occupy a smaller corner of my picture than my real values dawned one day shortly after I had closed this journal, this address to my now ex-husband—not, I think, entirely coincidentally.

I woke to sunlight, sat up suddenly, said decisively, "I don't have to live here any more!"

The clarity of it. The authenticity of it. The audaciousness. I can climb out of Noel's pocket completely, not just half-way out, sliding my eyes from left to right to left in case the bogey man is lurking, but right out. Away from his cattle, for which I was assuming more and more responsibility. Away from the hectares of pasture, which bore now, along with the thistles, only the ghost of my story of a rainforest retreat for the many. A hungry ghost. Eating my time, my energy, almost all of my money, in my determination to put flesh on its bones. And it had started to happen that each time I stepped out there, checking water levels for a spurious beef industry or else bristling from the waist up with weed-killing gear, an image of Noel withdrawn to the Gold Coast would form before me, and I was not smiling at him.

Associations from the previous four years rubbed shoulders for the entire length of our very long driveway. Memories held conversations across the paddocks and inside the bathroom waste-bin. The insistent fingers of my aspirations for that place plucked at me daily.

I had not wanted forty hectares anyway. I had left Sydney with modest visions of ... three? ... four? Then someone showed Noel the money in beef.

Our best chance of remaining the friends that we are, I told him during the evening that followed that dawn, is to sell this place, divide the proceeds in half—I'm entitled to that I think—and I'll raise whatever extra I need to get a smaller place of my own. Where? Near Mullumbimby, where I feel more at home than in cattle country, where I have more friends, where I have two teaching jobs. But my place will still be our place. It will still be your second home, I told him. I would want that. Jack would want that.

He understood. He was not happy, but he understood.

He made efforts to dissuade me, but he understood. His sadness was a by-product of my growth, just as mine had been of his. There was more letting go to be done.

For Jack the sadness was underscored by lack of understanding. Why would the Best Man In The World and The Best Woman In The World not stay together? But with the child's largesse he entered into the search for another home and said on first seeing the property we finally bought, "This place is filthy, Mum!" Mentally removing myself from the youthful torture of the language, I agreed. It is a place I could make my mandala, one with many windows for Jack. He and Ben have already christened the meditation room a squash court. Closer to his friends, he can bike to town.

Four separate timber buildings in four hectares of mostly rainforest, some paddocks for the ponies, water pumped from the river, it stands for an independence of spirit that I do not yet possess. The situation is bigger than me. Yet I know the energy for it will come. Already this energy has made itself felt: by the fact that there was not even one ripple in the hazardous waters of negotiating my first mortgage. By the phone call, the day after my offer on the place was accepted, from a fellow meditator, a stranger to me who said joyfully, when I told her the location of the new property, "I built that house!" By taking my anxiety to make things happen and transforming it into certainty that I was on my true path.

I have already held the first meditation retreat here. Chittaprabha came from Sydney to lead it. We accommodated a dozen women, including the original owner, who commented, "It's wonderful to see the place being put to such good use!" The response to Chittaprabha's clarity, to her as an example of living the dharma in our complex Western daily lives, was an inspiration. "Will you be back?" they asked. Yes.

How simple.

How very, very appropriate.

And yet ... How did this happen? When not so long ago what Noel and I both feared most was the pain a traditional separation might inflict upon Jack. Some people have been willing to answer that question, most in terms I can only describe as highly subjective. Who was it that pointed out, "Objectivity is the name men have given to their subjectivity?". Whoever it was—and I will assume it was a woman—she was, looking at it subjectively of course, quite right. Objectivity tries to put distance between the object observed and the observer. To divide them. To say they have nothing to do with one another. This, as both the quantum physicists and the Old Wives of the Tales know, would lead to a universe of total non-interaction. An enclosed system. A symmetrical universe. A universe where nothing happened.

Clearly though things do happen. And they happen because we are in a constant state of connection with one another, and with other phenonomena. A child could tell us that. Still we grown-ups insist upon putting up Pink Floyd's Walls, and defending them against those who would find a chink in our point of view.

How would the archetypal macho male define his degree of separation vis-a-vis my marriage breakup? *That poor bastard Noel! Slaving to please her for near on seventeen years, doesn't even TOUCH another flaming woman, and what does she do? Turns her flaming back on him when the poor bloke's hot for it. I mean. A man's gotta keep fit, eh?*

Or the other extreme, the radical, separatist feminist? *The silly cow. Typical mainstream female, even if she does dress herself up in geriatric radicalism. She's smiling far too much. Out to please everybody. Her darling Noel used her according to the patriarchal world-view: like a commodity. Now she's spent. He's spent her. She's the only one that doesn't know it.*

Or someone who sees everything in terms of sex? *Frigid. That's her problem. What do you expect from a woman who never even masturbated? Look at what she* didn't *do with her early boyfriends! She's all up in her head. Out past Pluto with a book on theoretical physics.*

Or in terms of age? *She was seven years older than him. He traded her in for a newer model. That's all.*

Or a reluctant father? *Women! They get their babies from you, then it's goodbye honeymoon.*

Or a professional homemaker? *Men! She kept a beautiful home for him, loved him, gave him a fine son, remained faithful to him, even wrote him poems ...*

Or a psychotherapist? *I'd like to know more about her father telling her to dry between her legs when she was seven years old.*

Or a pop astrologer? *He's a Gemini. He wants two of everything. She's Pisces. Sentimental to a fault.*

Or a menopausal woman? *Ratbag! Just when a woman most needs to be appreciated, not necessarily fucked, just appreciated, he tells her she's not up to scratch any more.*

Or a woman who runs with the wolves? *She's beginning to live her myth, finally. He will learn from that, he has already started. They may yet have work to do together.*

Or a female Western Buddhist? *She rediscovered a sense of her own completeness, and, like the rest of us, lost her man as a result.*

Or a supremely non-separate Zen Buddhist? *Whether their relationship crumbles or not is less important than what is learned ...*

None of these viewpoints cancels out any of the others. There is truth in each of them, and all of them together are not the only truths. To dwell with only one or even a few of them is to ignore the ambiguity around sex and marriage — and marriage, let's face it, has always been subject to fashion.

The idea that everybody has a right to romantic love started (or at least first became noticeable in retrospect) somewhere within the labyrinthine plots of Victorian novels.

Then newspapers, and in this century radio, cinema, TV,

the paperback and the pop music industry all seized on love as a saleable item. And what smoother way to sell a product than to make your potential customers feel incomplete without it? Marriage-for-all was packaged and sold to us as absolutely and thoroughly as only the modern media can package and sell. So that by the time I came along in 1944 it was deemed no strange thing to see our literary and popular heroes and heroines putting all their energy into making one another miserable either because they were not married, or because they were.

To my child's awakened eyes, miracles abounded. But clearly, judging by the purgatory it appeared to inflict, "being in love" was not one of them. That awareness began to change for me when puberty coincided with Hollywood's most expensive out-gushing of romantic tripe to date. Still, I managed to keep holding up my personal crucifix against the bad magic of *Seven Brides For Seven Brothers* until I was well past the traditional old-maid stage.

Noel's enthusiasm for our union nearly twenty years ago swept me off my feet. What an apt term that is. My falling in love was, after all, a state of sensing my individual inadequacy. My feet, which had supported me well enough among herds of African elephants and in classrooms-full of French delinquents, I had now conferred upon this man: let him take the steps for us both. I gave him my male-ness. Projected it onto him.

And so, in my incompleteness, I became part of the consensus. I was definable: a wife, and later, a mother. The words "wife" and "mother" may have drawn a quiet respect in previous eras, but this century's social, political and economic discourse, a discourse so very public, so very competitive, has had the effect of debasing language. As corporations rather than people have more and more to do with shaping our children's understanding, the terms "wife" and "mother" become increasingly synonymous with one-who-smiles-at-the-oat-bran-packet. Thus to be called wife or mother robs me of my individuality. However, paradox is always at play. Although the use of words may plunder my individuality, the use of words may also illuminate the place where my true self is hidden. Which is why I kept this journal. Where there is honesty, every word written is a blow struck for personal freedom.

In the writing of it, I was alone. But very rarely lonely. Because in writing it, I was finally with myself. To the earnest friend I saw recently who baled me up in the corner of the party with his undoubtedly genuine concern for the people of Rwanda, my inward endeavours seemed silly, scheming, self-serving.

He did not wish to make the connection that I had made, that regardless of how anxious we profess to be over humanity in general, it is in hurting people in our little daily lives that war finds its incubation. My quest is to learn to avoid inflicting such hurts, not because I think I *should* be peaceable and fear sanctions if I am not, but because I like the results of compassion.

My friend of the social conscience turned his back upon me.

Left me.

Left me with the enormity of quite ordinary things.

Like breaking promises to children.

Like leaving your family because it is no longer "ideal".

Like turning sex into a commodity.

From the furnace that sex makes of our bodies we bring fires into being that leave us spent. The act has spent us. The act is bigger than us both, can transport us beyond ourselves, beside ourselves, into realms bordering the mystical. No wonder sex is popular. We do not understand it with our minds. We do not want to understand it with our minds. By whose understanding might we attach labels to the magic that creates life, to the phoenix that continues to rise?

My relentless drive towards integrity made me recognise

that menopause had turned me away from the need for sexual congress and indeed for "a man". And my gradually increasing willingness to ring the changes, to discuss what was happening to me, to my body and to my life, combined with Noel's honesty to leave me sitting amongst the bits and pieces of my marriage, wondering which to leave lying in the ashes.

I was not alone. Smoke was rising all around me from the fires of marriages altered by female Change. In other words, I was not the only one of my peers to have gone off sex during her menopause. By which I mean normal Western several-times-a-week sex; few that I know would eschew it to the extent of wanting total prohibition. Indeed no. The occasional flight beyond our fully-clothed selves still gets talked about. And I stress *occasional*. A quota? A statistic? Oh dear. Pin us down then, as we sit in agreement over cups of herbal tea, to ... say ... maybe ... once in a while ... every few weeks ... every few months. But not a *daily* concern. Not a *daily* chore. Not that constant niggling domestic anxiety.

Why I am harping on sex? Is this book, then, about sex? After all, it opened with my pubescent longings for Rhett Butler. Is this *still* some sort of longing on my part? Just now, as the bud of my little child's feeling for *all* the world—not just for possible male protectors—just as that bud frosted by adulthood appears to be finally blossoming, I find it very difficult to answer that question. What I *can* say with confidence is that the story our society tells of sex is so well-packaged, so convincing, that in playing it down as I did, I left a vacancy in Noel's life much bigger than the one I had actually filled.

To what extent was my playing down of the sexual partnership hormonal? To what extent a result of my being with myself and beginning to see the possibilities of my own vision? To what extent was it both? I read somewhere that the greatest fool can ask more questions than the wisest person can answer. So once again I will be wise and say I don't know. Which also means I don't know whether or not this book is about sex.

To pretend that I know would be a lie. And what I *do* know is that for me menopause has meant that nothing matters so much as honesty. Integrity. I can't be fifty years old and a liar. What shame! The lies of my youth were as much from ignorance as they were from expediency, old enemies that I am learning to recognise before they have a chance to wreak too much havoc. My doors are open, and the winds that gust through them were fanned by Noel's courage and grace in sharing as much as he did about his careful, if unconscious, programme to ensure my dependence on him early in our marriage.

For two years I had been steering against him because he would not recognise his role in relegating my Dreaming to the bourgeois comfort zone. Then, suddenly, he turned and started to see the things I had always suspected of being there. Ironic? Had I not fallen into the marriage trap in the first place I might never have been in a material position to follow my Land-and-Community-Dreaming. But what price such a hollow speculation? The universe is not twice given.

Enough time has now elapsed that I grow used to his parallel company. We look across the divide as friends. No longer the talk of "perhaps". No longer the "if we become lovers again". The HRT did not live up to its reputation. It failed to make me jump him. Or anybody else. Loaded with oestrogen, I continued to teach English, kill weeds, meditate, hold my pee till I got to the toilet, and talk talk talk with the thousand-and-one women that have entered my life.

I stayed on the therapy for about six months before starting to nibble smaller and smaller bits off the pills each day as a way of weaning myself off it. It worked. It helped. I had no PMT in that crucial and sensitive time of transition.

I have had no bleeding since stopping the therapy. Perhaps it's all over. No more eggs? I've said that before somewhere. I'll make no more wild claims. Suffice to say my current daily nod in the direction of my menopause inclines mainly towards my juicer and my diet in general.

I still haven't had a hot flush. Something tells me I never will. Something tells me it is over, this time of physical malaise and mental confusion.

My body is older, looks older. But my heart is young. It has found again its mislaid purpose. I still sometimes cry for my lost "family", but I feel the mourning is almost complete. Because it has to be. It has to be, so that I can continue. I now look to a life either with Noel's friendship or without it. Either way it will happen of its own accord. Our idealised pictures of one another have been taken down. The manipulation inherent in being "married" has ended and the discussion now centres upon how best to be not "married".

People say to me, "He'll stop being your friend soon enough. Soon as you find yourself another man".

I say to them, "Maybe".

I am different now. I may never "find myself another man", in the sense that I found myself Noel. In the sense that he and Jan are now together. When I first met her at the renovated barn of the old property — Noel did not sell it, he let the house, moved his gear to the barn, and raised a loan to buy me out — I said, by way of introduction, "I don't know which of us feels stranger, but I'm glad this is happening". She concurred.

My childhood conditioning has not been eliminated, can never be eliminated. But I can stop paying attention to it. I can loosen the guy-ropes that tied me to it for years. My meditation fosters the conditions necessary for me to see what is hidden behind my eyes, to see into the reality that love and compassion always, *always* triumph. Not without pain, of course, not without suffering; but there is far more pain and suffering in hatred and in war.

There are gaps in my sense of wholeness, and through them enter fears—like my recent words to Noel, prompted because we see less of him now that he has two homes as well as ours, now that he is living *his* version of freedom: "It's me who is bringing up Jack", I said. Accusing. Fearful. "That's right", he replied, disarming me with his agreement, "and you're doing a great job."

A great job? Well. The job I most feared to be left alone with. The job that haunts me all the way home after I have seen them at the street corners, hardly older than Jack, with pins through their noses, their lips, their eyebrows. Our feral children. They are a judgement upon us. We are responsible.

And we are responsible for their music. Listen to it. Listen to the lyrics. They may throw all our conventions in our faces, but they are still going ga-ga over the equivalent of "Tea For Two". They are all looking for love embodied in some*one*. The model we have constructed is exclusive. It has nothing to do with love, which, as Shakespeare put it, does not alter "when it alteration finds". Love recognises change. It knows impermanence. Deny impermanence and you may as well blow raspberries at a force of nature.

Our children need another model. One based on community. On co-operation rather than exclusiveness. Outside the economic prison that speaks only of survival, says nothing of life.

But there. I shall do what I can. If in the absence of his father my son is stalked by his own masculinity, it is possible that some of the gaps in my wholeness will be healed over by what I have to offer him. All that I have to offer him is what I know as a woman: retain your good heart, my son; it is your manhood, it is your courage, it is your fearlessness to be who you are.

Then, perhaps not until you are much older, when your eyes meet mine across the boundless complexities of life, then, perhaps, you will understand.